THE DALLAS DOCTORS' DIET

THE DALLAS DOCTORS' DIET

Sandra Breithaupt
H. Wayne Agnew, M.D.

McGRAW-HILL BOOK COMPANY
New York   St. Louis   San Francisco   Toronto
Hamburg   Mexico

Copyright © 1983 by Sandra Breithaupt and H. Wayne Agnew, M.D.

1 2 3 4 5 6 7 8 9 F G R F G R 8 7 6 5 4 3

ISBN 0-07-007447-X

LIBRARY OF CONGRESS CATALOGING IN PUBLICATION DATA

Breithhaupt, Sandra.
  The Dallas doctors' diet.

  Includes index.
  1. Reducing diets. I. Agnew, H. Wayne. II. Title.
RM222.2.B73   613.2'5   82–24877

Book design by Judy Allan

To Justin, who has loved me both fat and thin, and who understands and is there for me now that I have decided to get everyone else thin. And to Betty, my True Thin friend, who gave me the inspiration for it all.   S. B.

To Wanda, who has given me support through thick and thin. And to my patients, whose participation and cooperation contributed greatly to this book.   H. W. A.

ACKNOWLEDGMENTS

WE WISH TO express our deepest gratitude to the doctors who shared their weight-loss story in this book. Not one of them did so for personal recognition, as each has more than enough; they did so because they wish to help others conquer obesity in a responsible, healthy manner. Doctors Bane, Daniel, Mendelson, Pirtle, Reitman and Wilson are fine, dedicated and caring men, and we are proud that they agreed to associate themselves with this project.

We would also like to acknowledge our deep appreciation to the three thousand plus people who have taken the Naturally Slim course. From their case histories we were able to compile the invaluable data on weight loss that is included in this book. Each of them has proven that what *you*, the reader, will be doing, has worked successfully for them.

We also wish to thank Terry Garrity, whose loving support, professional expertise and wisdom gave this book wings; and Theron Raines, our agent, whose dedication to this project went far beyond the usual obligations of an agent to an author.

CONTENTS

PREFACE

THE
DALLAS
DOCTORS

SEVEN OVERWEIGHT DALLAS doctors elected to try personally the new diet in this book and have given their permission for us to share their dieting experiences with you. The doctors are:

H. WAYNE AGNEW, M.D.
(co-author)

Dr. Agnew, a native Texan, is in private practice in obstetrics and gynecology in Arlington, Texas, just outside of Dallas. He is a graduate of the University of Texas Medical Branch, interned at William Beaumont Army

Hospital, and took his residency in obstetrics and gynecology at Parkland Memorial Hospital in Dallas, Texas. He is a member of the American Medical Association, the Texas Medical Association, the American College of Obstetrics and Gynecology, the American Fertility Society, the American Society of Gynecological Laparoscopists, and a Diplomate of the American Board of Obstetrics and Gynecology.

Dr. Agnew is married to his college sweetheart, Wanda, and they have three children, Michael, Sheryl and Scott.

Dr. Agnew's weight at the beginning of the Dallas Doctors' Diet program: 246½ pounds.

JERRY W. BANE, M.D.

Dr. Bane is a graduate of the University of Texas Southwestern Medical School. He did his residency in General Surgery at the University of Mississippi Medical Center. Dr. Bane is a Diplomate of the American Board of Surgery, a Fellow of the American College of Surgeons, and has the distinction of being a member of Phi Beta Kappa.

Dr. Bane and his wife, Marsha, have two children, Marc and Margaret. Both Marsha and Margaret are graduates of the Naturally Slim program.

Dr. Bane's weight at the beginning of the Dallas Doctors' Diet program: 191 pounds.

CLIFTON R. DANIEL, M.D.

Dr. Daniel graduated from the University of Texas Southwestern Medical School, did his internship at Parkland Memorial Hospital in Dallas, his residency in Pathology at the same institution. Dr. Daniel is a Diplomate of the American Board of Clinical, Anatomical and Dermatopathology, is a Fellow of the College of American Pathologists and the American Society of Clinical Pathologists, and is a member of Alpha Omega Alpha.

Dr. Daniel's wife, Myrtle, although she is a True Thin, attended each diet class with her husband to lend support and learn how to adapt this new way of eating to the family's meal schedules.

Dr. and Mrs. Daniel have two teenage boys, William and Andy.

Dr. Daniel's weight at the beginning of the Dallas Doctors' Diet program: 200 pounds.

MICHAEL MENDELSON, M.D.

Dr. Mendelson is a graduate of George Washington University Medical School and did his internship and residency at the same institution. Dr. Mendelson holds a Fellowship in Gastroenterology from the University of Colorado Medical School. He is a Diplomate of the American Board of Internal Medicine and the American Board of Gastroenterology, and a member of the American College of Physicians, the American Gastroenterological Association, and the American Society of Gastrointestinal Endoscopy.

Dr. Mendelson's wife, Carole, is a biochemist, and they have four children, Laurie, Sandra, Andrew and Barbara.

Dr. Mendelson's weight at the beginning of the program: 224 pounds.

WILLIAM PIRTLE, M.D.

Dr. Pirtle graduated from Baylor College of Medicine in Houston and did his internship at Baylor University Hospitals in Dallas. His postgraduate training in General Surgery was received at the Veterans Administration Hospital in Dallas and the John Peter Smith Hospital in Fort Worth. He is a member of the American Academy of Family Physicians.

Dr. Pirtle and his wife, Joyce, have one son.

Dr. Pirtle's weight at the beginning of the program: 217 pounds.

SANFORD REITMAN, M.D.

Dr. Reitman graduated from the University of Alabama Medical College, did his internship at Philadelphia Naval Hospital, his residency in Radiology at San Diego Naval Hospital, Isotope Engineering at Scripps Institute, U.C.L.A., and Nuclear Medicine at the National Naval Medical Center in Bethesda, Maryland. He also holds a fellowship in radiologic pathology from the Armed Forces Institute of Pathology, Walter Reed Hospital, Bethesda, Maryland.

Dr. Reitman is a Diplomate of the American Board of Radiology, a Fellow of the National Institute of Health, Institute of Neurological Diseases and Blindness (Neuro-Anatomy), a member of the American College of Radiology, and a member or fellow of numerous other medical societies.

Dr. Reitman and his wife, Margie, have three children, Lauren, Deborah and Mitchell.

Dr. Reitman's weight at the beginning of the program: 198 pounds.

JACK WILSON, D.D.S.

Dr. Wilson is a graduate of Baylor College of Dentistry in Dallas. He is a member of the American Dental Association, the Texas Dental Association and the Academy of General Dentistry.

Dr. Wilson and his wife, Betty, have two sons, Andy and Eric.

Dr. Wilson's weight at the beginning of the Dallas Doctors' Diet program: 237½ pounds.

INTRODUCTION

WHEN ALL THE DIETS FAILED ME

I AM NOW, and have been for a number of years, a thin person . . . but I wasn't always blessed with a naturally slim body.

I was a plump baby, a roly-poly youngster, a heavy teenager and, when I wasn't starving myself, an obese adult. I have spent nearly a third of my life obsessed with food—craving it, rejecting it; stuffing myself, denying myself. Looking back on my fat years I realize I spent thousands of hours thinking about food, talking about food, reading about food, shopping for food, preparing food, eating food and suffering real torment because of food. For despite the fact that I am an intelligent, strong-willed and disciplined person, the end results of every

1

one of my many battles to control my weight were always
the same:

self-loathing	100%
guilt	100%
anguish	100%
suffering during dieting	100%
permanent weight loss	0%

Does this sound all too familiar to you?

I embarked upon my first diet at the age of sixteen. I
simply stopped eating—except for one small apple a day.
My parents forbade me to experiment with any extreme
diet regimens in the future. And to make sure I didn't
do anything foolish, my mother asked our family doctor
to give me a safe, sensible diet to help me shed my "baby
fat." He prescribed amphetamines (in the 1950's such
prescriptions were handed out liberally to people fighting
obesity). Amphetamines did, indeed, curb my appetite
and help me lose weight, but as soon as each prescription
was exhausted, the pounds would rapidly return. I knew
there had to be a better solution to obesity than addictive
drugs, and so in the 1960's I began experimenting with,
and failed at, every fad diet I came across. Remember
Dr. Taller's safflower-oil diet? The Air Force diet? The
grapefruit-and-egg diet? The 600-calorie-a-day diet? The
brown-rice diet? The rainbow diet? I tried them all, plus
the magazine diets, the latest best-selling diet books and
the theories and regimens of the diet clubs such as Weight
Watchers and T.O.P.S. that were becoming popular. I
even consulted a famous bariatric physician in New York
and a diet "guru" in California. All these diets worked
. . . while I was on them; but my weight always sneaked

back as soon as I stopped starving and again began eating the foods that were important to me.

Eventually I ran out of new diet theories to test on my protesting body. In total, complete frustration, one day I put my fork and my head down on the table and cried. I could not eat another hard-boiled egg, another piece of broiled chicken or another salad with imitation dressing.

All the diets had failed me.

And worn out with years of punishing myself mentally, emotionally and physically, I said to myself, "Sandra, life is too short to spend it making yourself miserable with apparently unrealistic goals. You have done your best, but the fat has won. You're just going to have to learn to accept the fact that 35 or so extra pounds have apparently taken up permanent residence on your body!"

I vowed never to diet again, but I did remain intensely curious about why some people could eat anything they wanted to and never gain an ounce, while seemingly everything I ate went instantly to fat. Were the thin people of this world born with more efficient metabolisms? Did they eat differently? Were they immune to the pleasures of high-calorie foods? Were their appetite control signals more active than mine? Did they inherit thin body cells and I fat ones?

In my spare time I studied the eating habits of perennially skinny people—the True Thins of this world. They did indeed eat *differently* from fat people like myself, but oddly enough they didn't eat *less* than I did. And they seemed to enjoy food as much as I did. What was the secret to their ability to eat anything they liked, when they liked, without gaining a pound?

One night . . . by chance . . . something a True Thin

said in passing made me realize that the answer to getting and staying thin was within my grasp. I had just heard *the crucial piece of information that would change me from a chronically overweight person into a True Thin forever!*

Using my discovery of the truly surprising answer to permanent slimness, in 1971 I lowered my weight from 145 pounds to 104 pounds and, more impressively, *kept* off the 41 pounds that had been my nemesis for so many years.

I was overjoyed!

Naturally my overweight friends in Shreveport, where I live, wanted to know what new miracle diet I had used to get thin and, in an informal way, I guided them through the same simple program I had designed for myself— and they effortlessly lost weight too.

Definitely my diet worked for me and my overweight friends, but would it be successful with strangers? By a lucky coincidence at that time (1975) I was training to be a transactional analysis psychotherapist, and as part of that training I had to form a therapy group. I didn't really feel ready to work with the severely ill, but I did have great empathy for obese people, and so I gathered together a group of fat people who were motivated to solve their weight problems, and by using transactional analysis methods in combination with my new diet discovery, my group lost their extra pounds as easily and cheerfully as I had.

I was very excited. My diet wasn't a fluke, I really had discovered how to help fat people become thin! Word of my success spread quickly around Shreveport and suddenly I was inundated with requests for weight counseling. I formed several more groups and from my experiences with them was able to design a professional weight-loss course, which in 1977 was incorporated under the trade name "Naturally Slim." Today, I have instructors working under my supervision throughout Louisiana and Texas, teaching people how to become naturally slim forever. And I am very proud to be able to say that *Naturally Slim produces better long-term weight-loss results than any other diet program in the world.*

In this book I have taken the key weight-losing elements of my six-week course and condensed them into a simple how-to program that you can do at home so that you, too, can become the True Thin person of your dreams. I promise you that on my diet you can lose your ugly, unhealthy extra pounds, and without suffering the horrors and humiliations of standard dieting. For the Dallas Doctors' Diet is *not* a deprivation diet.

Remember, my program is based on an entirely new concept of how to win the fight against obesity, so on this diet you will experience:

- no hunger pangs
- no waiting for days for a pound's loss
- no freak treatments such as hormone injections, diet pills and other pharmacological aids
- no calorie counting
- no food weighing
- no yo-yoing
- no abstinence from liquor
- no uncomfortable physical side effects
- no emotional mood swings
- no having to avoid social functions featuring gourmet foods
- no feeling of being different because "I'm on a diet again."

I realize you are curious about what my revolutionary new diet concept is, but before we begin, you need to know how my "Naturally Slim" course became "The Dallas Doctors' Diet." Let me introduce my co-author and the medical consultant for this book: Dr. Wayne Agnew.

Like Sandra Breithaupt, I am no stranger to obesity. I too, was a "plump" baby, but in Texas in 1934, the year I was born, that was considered good. Fat babies were thought to be the ideal. In fact, my mother felt I was such a perfect baby that she entered me in a Sears, Roebuck contest to find the most beautiful baby in America, and I was a finalist. I still have an engraved cup and some yellowed newspaper clippings to prove it. But while pudginess may be an asset in babies, when I reached school age I discovered that the world thinks thin people are more acceptable than fat ones. I was what my mother fondly called "stocky" and thanks to the good ol' Texas cooking I got at home I stayed "stocky." So did my whole family.

I paid a cruel price for all that good food my family lovingly stuffed into me, for hardly a day passed but that some kids in school ridiculed me, and I got beat up a lot because I was so fat that I was a sitting duck for the gangs. When we had to do square dancing in the gymnasium Dolores Hemple, who was the prettiest and most popular girl in school, would point at my rear end and laugh at me because my butt jiggled when I skipped around the circles.

I was so miserable that when I entered junior high I took desperate measures. I had never heard of diets, so, like Sandra, I fasted.

My parents got worried and even threatened to take me to see Titus Harris, a prominent psychiatrist; he was chairman of the department at the medical school in Galveston.

But I wouldn't listen. I refused to eat for weeks until I finally got so thin my collar bones stuck out, and then I went back to eating again.

Peer pressure can be vicious. In my case it bothered me so much I was willing to starve myself to win peer approval.

The only time of my life I can remember when I did not have to fight the scales was during my years in medical school, interning, and during my residency in obstetrics/gynecology. In those days, I was kept on the run and had so little time for sleeping and eating that I didn't have a chance to put on any weight. For instance, when I was doing my residency at Parkland Hospital in Dallas, I was up all night—24 hours on, 24 hours off—and we might have as many as 25, 35 or even 45 deliveries during a shift; some of these mothers would roll right in off the street never having even been to a clinic, much less a private doctor, so there were very few simple deliveries. I was responsible for all those births. I had students under me, but because I was in charge it was always a stressful 24 hours. I *lost* weight then.

My weight started to creep back about fourteen years ago, when I went into private practice. The busier I got, the more I rewarded myself with food, which was easy to come by. My office nurses were always bringing in some goody or other they had cooked, the hospital nurses had big boxes of candy at their stations and there were always those tempting doughnuts and coffee waiting for me any time I wanted to take a break after surgery or rounds. So it's not surprising that every year I had a steady weight gain interspersed with a little diet from time to time. I tried a number of diets—one I got out of the medical journals, the Carnation, the Scarsdale, Weight Watchers. And, like

Sandra, once I got off each diet I promptly regained all the weight I had lost.

All diets I knew about that were safe were bearable for a short while only. None of them tackled the problem of keeping your weight down when you returned to eating regular foods and meals, and none of them took individual hunger patterns and food tastes into consideration. That's why I was particularly alert to the fact that my sister Emily wasn't on one of her usual fad diets when she showed up in Dallas for our annual Thanksgiving family gathering in 1980. She was 30 pounds thinner, but that in itself wasn't unusual, for Emily was always dieting and then regaining every pound she'd lost plus a few more pounds, but what was different, I realized, about Emily this time was *how* she was eating. To put it bluntly, it had never been Emily's style to pick and choose when confronted with a big buffet table full of food. In fact, she was famous for taking some of everything and eating it all, as if it were her sacred duty. But here she was all of a sudden selecting only her favorite foods and eating them like she was a gourmet, and looking contented throughout the whole meal. I had never seen a diet like that, one where you could eat nearly every kind of food and lose weight.

Since I was still searching for a healthy lifetime way of staying thin for both myself and my chronically overweight patients, I arranged to meet the woman who had worked such wonders with my sister. I flew to Shreveport and consulted with Sandra Breithaupt; and I was so impressed with her theories on weight loss that I decided to make myself a test case.

I began the Naturally Slim course with 247 pounds on my 6-foot frame and at the end of six weeks had dropped to 215 pounds, despite the fact that I continued to eat all of my favorite, usually fattening foods. Since then I have lost another 25 pounds and kept them off. In fact, I think that was what impressed me most about Sandra's diet— she had verified statistics that showed that 80% of the people who had taken her course had not regained their lost weight. As a physician, I am aware that very few people are able to keep the weight off that they lose on diets. Figures of people maintaining weight loss vary from 5% to 15%, depending upon the diet.

Obviously, there is something wrong with most diet programs if only a tiny percentage of people can achieve long-term weight-loss success. I believe the reason that all the diets failed Sandra, me and most other people who tried them is that they were artificial ways of eating, ways that the human body rejected, just as it rejects foreign substances.

Sandra Breithaupt is not a physician, but she instinctively hit upon a basic truth: allow your body to function in the efficient way it was designed to function, and it will heal itself. In the case of obesity, which I consider to be a disease, if you remove the abnormal system of food ingestion that you have forced upon your protesting body and restore it to normal food intake patterns, the body will cure itself of obesity.

I was the first Dallas doctor to discover Sandra Breithaupt and her ingenious new way of losing weight. I became convinced that her program was an excellent one, but I wanted verification from experts I respected. In 1981 I invited several of my chronically overweight colleagues to give Naturally Slim a try to see if they could duplicate my success. I also wanted to pick their fine medical brains about the safety and practical application of this diet. You will read in this book how these Dallas doctors did on the Naturally

Slim program. For myself, I say this: I feel that this diet is the best one I have ever come across in my entire medical career. I recommend it to all my overweight patients who seek my advice on how to lose weight healthily, happily and forever, and I recommend it to you for your consideration.

1

THE DALLAS DOCTORS' AND YOUR EATING PROFILES

OVERWEIGHT PEOPLE DON'T like to think about their eating habits, for knowledge of how much, how often and what you eat daily is likely to produce strong feelings of guilt and lack of self-worth. The last thing I want to do is make you feel miserable about your food habits; I think diets that preach or assign blame are cruel and destructive, but if you are going to succeed at this, your very last diet, you are going to have to become aware of your present eating patterns so that you can learn what is important to you and what is not.

Everybody has tried to fool with your food before, telling you you can't eat this favorite food or that one if you want to be thin. I am not going to do that. I realize you like the foods you are eating now, even love many of them, and you like them prepared in ways that are pleasing to *you*—perhaps fried or raw, or basted with lovely sauces, or breaded. I guarantee you, I will not try to get you to change your food tastes. I *am* going to urge you to change your *pattern* of food intake, and to do that you will have to take control of when and how you eat.

To exercise intelligent control you must become knowledgeable about your present eating patterns so that you can make decisions about the kinds of changes you can live with.

At the end of this chapter you will find a form. It is YOUR EATING PROFILE form. Please fill it out as candidly and completely as possible and then study your answers. The meaning of your responses will become clear to you in the succeeding chapters.

Before you fill out your personal profile, study the Dallas doctors' profiles. You will notice that each doctor has his own highly individual food tastes and ways of eating. Some of these will change as they progress through the first weeks of the diet, but none of the doctors will suffer feelings of deprivation, frustration, guilt or depression.

Neither will you, if you learn enough about your food needs to meet those needs intelligently.

Note: If you do not wish anyone to see the answers to YOUR EATING PROFILE, I suggest that you photocopy the form, fill it out at a time when you are alone, and then keep it in a private place. None of the questions is unduly personal, but I am aware that you may be supersensitive to prying eyes, thanks to years of living in a society that has told you that overweight people are weak, self-destructive and self-indulgent if they eat any foods that are not low calorie. Such attitudes may have forced you into hiding your real eating habits from others and even yourself. For instance, I used to have "amnesia" about the little afternoon pick-me-ups I ate to get me through until dinnertime because I felt guilty whenever I ate outside of the "normal" three-meals-a-day schedule. I didn't realize that the fact that I needed a pick-me-up around 4:00 P.M. every day didn't mean that I was a spineless person, helpless to resist my relentless food cravings; instead, it was a clue to the fact that my food needs weren't being met.

After you have filled in your eating profile, turn to Chapter 2 to discover why the rich foods you like to eat don't have to be fattening.

YOUR EATING PROFILE

NAME *Wayne Agnew*   AGE *48* HEIGHT *6'*

PRESENT WEIGHT *247*   GOAL WEIGHT *190*

1. When did your weight problem begin? (Time and/or event) *birth*

2. List the last 4 diets you have tried, date, amount of weight lost, length of time.

Diet	Date	Amount Lost	Time on Diet
High protein	*1963*	*10 lbs.*	*1 month*
"	*1970*	*15 lbs.*	*2 months*
Scarsdale	*1979*	*20 lbs.*	*1 month*

3. If you were overweight as a child, what years? *always chubby (except in high school)*

4. What is the lowest you have weighed since age 23? *180*

5. On a normal weekend does your weight increase and, if so, how much? *yes*
   1–2 lbs.

6. On a weekend trip does your weight increase and, if so, how much? *yes*
   1–2 lbs.

7. Last year did you gain weight from Dec. 1 to Jan. 1? *yes* How much?
   5 lbs. How long did it take to lower your weight back to your Dec. 1
   weight? *3–4 weeks*

8. On the average, how much per year does your weight increase? *1–2 lbs.*

9. Is there a weight you cannot seem to go below no matter how hard you try? *not really* What is that weight? _____ When was the last time you weighed this? _____

10. Which of the following do you eat regularly?

√ Breakfast	_____ Mid-morning snack
√ Lunch	_____ Mid-afternoon snack
√ Dinner	_____ After-dinner snack

11. If you usually eat breakfast, or a "little something," about what time? *6–6:30* What do you eat and drink? *protein drink* _____

12. How often do you eat cereal during the week? Daily _____ 5 × week _____
    3 × week _____ 1 × week _____ seldom/never √

13. Circle those of the following you usually drink: (JUICES) . . . COLD DRINKS (SUGARED) . . (MILK) . . . (HEALTH DRINKS) . . . HOT/COLD CHOCOLATE . . . CUPS OF (SOUP) . . . MILK SHAKES

14. What are your favorite foods and snacks when you aren't dieting? *meat, potatoes, cheese, chips, food, food, food*

15. What low calorie foods do you really enjoy? *salads, fresh vegetables*

16. How often do you eat desserts? Daily _____ 5 × week _____ 3 × week _____
    1 × week _____ seldom/never √

17. Do you prefer soft or crunchy foods? _____ Both? _____ *yes* Spicy foods?

18. In order of preference, list kinds of bread you enjoy. *not a big bread eater*

_____

19. Are you a SLOW or (FAST) eater? Circle one.

20. Do you leave food on your plate? Yes _____ No ✓ *never* How often?

21. Do you ordinarily take seconds? Yes ✓ No _____ If yes, is it because you ✓ are still hungry _____ *usually do* urged to by parent, spouse, others

22. Do you eat more than usual or less when you are feeling:
more depressed *more* anxious
more nervous *less* excited
more angry *more* sad

23. As a child, did your parents encourage you to eat when you weren't hungry? *yes* Did they encourage you to clean your plate? *yes* Insist? *no*

24. Were you told you might get sick if you didn't eat at mealtime? *no*

25. When eating *at home* (and not dieting), which of the following do you usually eat at one meal? Salad ✓ Bread *no* Meat ✓ Vegetable ✓ Dessert *no*

26. When eating *out* (and not dieting), which of the following do you usually eat at one meal? Salad ✓ Bread ✓ Meat ✓ Vegetable ✓ Dessert *no*

27. Why do you believe you have a problem weighing what you want to weigh? _eat too much. I'm a card-carrying foodaholic._

28. Why do you believe some people stay at normal weight without dieting? _eat normally—they don't overeat._

29. Is there anyone in your family or do you have a friend who is a True Thin (someone who is normal weight and never diets)? Indicate the relationship (son, mother, husband, daughter, etc.) _son_

30. Do you take any medication that we should know about? _no_

31. Please make any additional comments about yourself or your lifestyle that you believe will enable us to help you in lowering your weight.

YOUR EATING PROFILE

NAME _Jerry Bane_   AGE _41_   HEIGHT _5'9"_

PRESENT WEIGHT _191_   GOAL WEIGHT _170_

1. When did your weight problem begin? (Time and/or event) _1966_

2. List the last 4 diets you have tried, date, amount of weight lost, length of time.

Diet	Date	Amount Lost	Time on Diet
Weight Watchers	_1966_	_1–5 lbs._	_1–2 months_
Self-styled (exercise)	_1966–78_	_3–5 lbs._	_off and on_

3. If you were overweight as a child, what years?

4. What is the lowest you have weighed since age 23? _165–170_

5. On a normal weekend does your weight increase and, if so, how much? _no_

6. On a weekend trip does your weight increase and, if so, how much? _no_

7. Last year did you gain weight from Dec. 1 to Jan. 1? _yes_ How much? _5 lbs._ How long did it take to lower your weight back to your Dec. 1 weight? _3 months_

18

8. On the average, how much per year does your weight increase? *5–10 lbs.*
Then lose?

9. Is there a weight you cannot seem to go below no matter how hard you try? *no* What is that weight? _____ When was the last time you weighed this? _____

10. Which of the following do you eat regularly?
    √ Breakfast   Mid-morning snack _____
    √ Lunch   Mid-afternoon snack _____
    √ Dinner   After-dinner snack _____

11. If you usually eat breakfast, or a "little something," about what time? *6:30* What do you eat and drink? *milk, cheese, toast*

12. How often do you eat cereal during the week? Daily _____ 5 × week _____
    3 × week _____ 1 × week √ seldom/never _____

13. Circle those of the following you usually drink: JUICES . . . COLD DRINKS (SUGARED)
    . . . (MILK) . . . HEALTH DRINKS . . . HOT/COLD CHOCOLATE . . . CUPS OF SOUP . . .
    MILK SHAKES

14. What are your favorite foods and snacks when you aren't dieting? *ice cream*

15. What low calorie foods do you really enjoy? *fruits and vegetables*

16. How often do you eat desserts? Daily √ 5 × week _____ 3 × week _____
    1 × week _____ seldom/never _____

19

17. Do you prefer soft or crunchy foods? _crunchy_ Both? _____ Spicy foods?

18. In order of preference, list kinds of bread you enjoy. _bread, rolls, biscuits, corn bread_

19. Are you a SLOW or (FAST) eater? Circle one.

20. Do you leave food on your plate? Yes _____ No √
How often?

21. Do you ordinarily take seconds? Yes √ No _____ If yes, is it because you _____ are still hungry √ usually do _____ urged to by parent, spouse, others _____

22. Do you eat more than usual or less when you are feeling:
    _____ depressed   _more_ anxious
    _____ nervous   _____ excited
    _____ angry   _____ sad

23. As a child, did your parents encourage you to eat when you weren't hungry?
    _____? Did they encourage you to clean your plate? _yes_ Insist? _no_

24. Were you told you might get sick if you didn't eat at mealtime? _no_

25. When eating _at home_ (and not dieting), which of the following do you usually eat at one meal? Salad _____ Bread √ Meat √ Vegetable √
Dessert √

26. When eating _out_ (and not dieting), which of the following do you usually eat

20

at one meal? Salad ___✓___ Bread ___✓___ Meat ___✓___ Vegetable ___✓___
Dessert ___✓___

27. Why do you believe you have a problem weighing what you want to weigh?
overeat

28. Why do you believe some people stay at normal weight without dieting?
metabolism, exercise

29. Is there anyone in your family or do you have a friend who is a True Thin
(someone who is normal weight and never diets)? Indicate the relationship (son,
mother, husband, daughter, etc.) *son*

30. Do you take any medication that we should know about? *no*

31. Please make any additional comments about yourself or your lifestyle that you
believe will enable us to help you in lowering your weight. *I run 6 to 10 miles*
daily

YOUR EATING PROFILE

NAME _Clifton Daniel_   AGE _____   HEIGHT _6'0"_

PRESENT WEIGHT _200_   GOAL WEIGHT _____

1. When did your weight problem begin? (Time and/or event) _College_

2. List the last 4 diets you have tried, date, amount of weight lost, length of time.

Diet	Date	Amount Lost	Time on Diet
Weight Watchers	_1970_	_35 lbs._	_several months_

3. If you were overweight as a child, what years? _8–12_

4. What is the lowest you have weighed since age 23? _160_

5. On a normal weekend does your weight increase and, if so, how much?
   2–5 lbs.

6. On a weekend trip does your weight increase and, if so, how much? _0_

7. Last year did you gain weight from Dec. 1 to Jan. 1? _yes_ How much?
   5 lbs. How long did it take to lower your weight back to your Dec. 1
   weight? _did not go down_

22

8. On the average, how much per year does your weight increase? _8 lbs._

9. Is there a weight you cannot seem to go below no matter how hard you try? _yes_ What is that weight? _168_ When was the last time you weighed this? _3 yrs. ago_

10. Which of the following do you eat regularly?

    _____ Breakfast   _____ Mid-morning snack

    _✓_ Lunch   _____ Mid-afternoon snack

    _✓_ Dinner   _✓_ After-dinner snack

11. If you usually eat breakfast, or a "little something," about what time? _7:00_ What do you eat and drink? _various foods, usually cereals_

12. How often do you eat cereal during the week? Daily _____ 5 × week _✓_ 3 × week _____ 1 × week _____ seldom/never _____

13. Circle those of the following you usually drink: JUICES. . . COLD DRINKS (SUGARED) . . . MILK . . . (HEALTH DRINKS). . . HOT/COLD CHOCOLATE . . CUPS OF SOUP . . . MILK SHAKES

14. What are your favorite foods and snacks when you aren't dieting? _salads, apples, bananas, fish, chicken, carrots, beans, potatoes, chips, coffee, apple pie_

15. What low calorie foods do you really enjoy? _fish, chicken_

16. How often do you eat desserts? Daily _✓_ 5 × week _____ 3 × week _____ 1 × week _____ seldom/never _____

23

17. Do you prefer soft or crunchy foods? _____ *crunchy* Both? _____ Spicy foods? _____

18. In order of preference, list kinds of bread you enjoy. *coarse breads—whole wheat, rye, pumpernickel, corn*

19. Are you a SLOW or (FAST) eater? Circle one.

20. Do you leave food on your plate? Yes _____ No _____ ✓ How often? *never*

21. Do you ordinarily take seconds? Yes ✓ No _____ If yes, is it because you _____ are still hungry ✓ usually do _____ urged to by parent, spouse, others

22. Do you eat more than usual or less when you are feeling:
    more depressed   *more* anxious
    " _____ nervous   " _____ excited
    " _____ angry   " _____ sad

23. As a child, did your parents encourage you to eat when you weren't hungry? *yes* Did they encourage you to clean your plate? *yes* Insist? *no*

24. Were you told you might get sick if you didn't eat at mealtime? *yes*

25. When eating *at home* (and not dieting), which of the following do you usually eat at one meal? Salad ✓ Bread ✓ Meat ✓ Vegetable ✓ Dessert ✓

26. When eating *out* (and not dieting), which of the following do you usually eat at one meal? Salad ✓ Bread ✓ Meat ✓ Vegetable ✓ Dessert _____

27. Why do you believe you have a problem weighing what you want to weigh? _They_
Inability to perceive satiety and distinguish hunger from other feelings

28. Why do you believe some people stay at normal weight without dieting? _They_
do not really care about food and eating

29. Is there anyone in your family or do you have a friend who is a True Thin
(someone who is normal weight and never diets)? Indicate the relationship (son,
mother, husband, daughter, etc.) _son_

30. Do you take any medication that we should know about? _no_

31. Please make any additional comments about yourself or your lifestyle that you
believe will enable us to help you in lowering your weight.

YOUR EATING PROFILE

NAME _Michael Mendelson_   AGE _____   HEIGHT _6'_

PRESENT WEIGHT _224_   GOAL WEIGHT _____

1. When did your weight problem begin? (Time and/or event) _10 years ago_

2. List the last 4 diets you have tried, date, amount of weight lost, length of time.

Diet	Date	Amount Lost	Time on Diet

3. If you were overweight as a child, what years? _____

4. What is the lowest you have weighed since age 23? _170_

5. On a normal weekend does your weight increase and, if so, how much? _no_

6. On a weekend trip does your weight increase and, if so, how much? _no_

7. Last year did you gain weight from Dec. 1 to Jan. 1? _no_ How much? _____
   How long did it take to lower your weight back to your Dec. 1 weight? _____

8. On the average, how much per year does your weight increase? _5 lbs._

9. Is there a weight you cannot seem to go below no matter how hard you try? _____

26

never tried What is that weight? _____ When was the last time you weighed this?

10. Which of the following do you eat regularly?

    Breakfast _____ Mid-morning snack _____

    Lunch _____ Mid-afternoon snack _____

    __✓__ Dinner _____ After-dinner snack __✓__ _before dinner_

11. If you usually eat breakfast, or a "little something," about what time? _____ What do you eat and drink? _____

12. How often do you eat cereal during the week? Daily _____ 5 × week _____ 3 × week _____ 1 × week _____ seldom/never __✓__

13. Circle those of the following you usually drink: (JUICES) . . (COLD DRINKS (SUGARED)) . . MILK . . . HEALTH DRINKS . . . (HOT/COLD CHOCOLATE) . . . CUPS OF SOUP . . . MILK SHAKES

14. What are your favorite foods and snacks when you aren't dieting? _Anything I can get my hands on. Usually take 2nd, 3rd and 4th servings. Ice cream; cookies_

15. What low calorie foods do you really enjoy? _____

16. How often do you eat desserts? Daily __✓__ 5 × week _____ 3 × week _____ 1 × week _____ seldom/never _____

17. Do you prefer soft or crunchy foods? _____ Both? __✓__ Spicy foods? __✓__

27

18. In order of preference, list kinds of bread you enjoy. _any kind_

19. Are you a SLOW or (FAST) eater? Circle one.

20. Do you leave food on your plate? Yes _____ No _never—clean other people's plates_ How often?

21. Do you ordinarily take seconds? Yes _✓_ No _____ If yes, is it because you _____ are still hungry _✓_ usually do _____ urged to by parent, spouse, others

22. Do you eat more than usual or less when you are feeling:

    _?_ depressed   _more_ anxious
    more nervous   _more_ excited
    _?_ angry   _?_ sad

23. As a child, did your parents encourage you to eat when you weren't hungry? _not sure_ Did they encourage you to clean your plate? _yes_ Insist? _not really_

24. Were you told you might get sick if you didn't eat at mealtime? _no_

25. When eating _at home_ (and not dieting), which of the following do you usually eat at one meal? Salad _____ Bread _____ Meat _____ Vegetable _✓_ Dessert _✓_

26. When eating _out_ (and not dieting), which of the following do you usually eat at one meal? Salad _✓_ Bread _✓_ Meat _✓_ Vegetable _____ Dessert _✓_

27. Why do you believe you have a problem weighing what you want to weigh?

progressively upward weight past 10–15 years; now up to 224 from usual 170 lbs. Clothes don't fit—wife UPSET!

28. Why do you believe some people stay at normal weight without dieting? *They probably control food intake more intelligently and don't allow stressful anxious moments to increase intake of food*

29. Is there anyone in your family or do you have a friend who is a True Thin (someone who is normal weight and never diets)? Indicate the relationship (son, mother, husband, daughter, etc.) *not in my family. Wife thin*

30. Do you take any medication that we should know about? *no*

31. Please make any additional comments about yourself or your lifestyle that you believe will enable us to help you in lowering your weight. *APPRECIATE FOOD*

YOUR EATING PROFILE

NAME *Bill Pirtle*

PRESENT WEIGHT ___217___   GOAL WEIGHT ___180___   AGE _52_ HEIGHT _6'0"_

1. When did your weight problem begin? (Time and/or event) _30 years ago_

2. List the last 4 diets you have tried, date, amount of weight lost, length of time.

Diet	Date	Amount Lost	Time on Diet
Scarsdale	*June 81*	*10*	*14 days*
Grapefruit	*Mar. 81*	*7*	*8 days*
Scarsdale	*Jan. 81*	*10*	*14 days*
Low Carbohydrate	*Mar. 79*	*18*	*4 weeks*

3. If you were overweight as a child, what years? _Ages 10–16_

4. What is the lowest you have weighed since age 23? _185_

5. On a normal weekend does your weight increase and, if so, how much? _yes_
   2 pounds

6. On a weekend trip does your weight increase and, if so, how much? _yes_
   2 pounds

7. Last year did you gain weight from Dec. 1 to Jan. 1? _yes_ How much?
   5 lbs. How long did it take to lower your weight back to your Dec. 1
   weight? _1 week_

30

8. On the average, how much per year does your weight increase? _none to 5_
   lbs.

9. Is there a weight you cannot seem to go below no matter how hard you try?
   yes What is that weight? _195_ When was the last time you weighed
   this? _June 1981_

10. Which of the following do you eat regularly?
    _____ Breakfast   Mid-morning snack
    _✓_ Lunch   Mid-afternoon snack
    _✓_ Dinner   After-dinner snack

11. If you usually eat breakfast, or a "little something," about what time?
    _8:00_ What do you eat and drink? _cereal and hot tea_

12. How often do you eat cereal during the week? Daily _____   5 × week _✓_
    3 × week _____   1 × week _____   seldom/never _____

13. Circle those of the following you usually drink: JUICES. . . COLD DRINKS (SUGARED)
    . . MILK. . . HEALTH DRINKS . . . HOT/COLD CHOCOLATE . . CUPS OF SOUP . . .
    MILK SHAKES

14. What are you favorite foods and snacks when you aren't dieting? _nachos and_
    Mexican food, cookies, bananas, fried potatoes

15. What low calorie foods do you really enjoy? _salads, diet drinks, certain vegeta-_
    bles (spinach, string beans, cabbage)

16. How often do you eat desserts? Daily _____   5 × week _____   3 × week

17. ___✓___ 1 × week _____ seldom/never _____ Both? ___✓___ Spicy _____
    Do you prefer soft or crunchy foods? *not necessarily*
    foods?

18. In order of preference, list kinds of bread you enjoy. *yeast rolls (do not eat
    bread much except in occasional sandwich)*

19. Are you a SLOW or (FAST) eater? Circle one.

20. Do you leave food on your plate? Yes _____ No ___✓___
    How often?

21. Do you ordinarily take seconds? Yes _____ No ___✓___ If yes, is it because
    you _____ are still hungry _____ usually do _____ urged to by parent,
    spouse, others

22. Do you eat more than usual or less when you are feeling:
    more depressed   *more* anxious
    " nervous   " excited
    " angry   " sad

23. As a child, did your parents encourage you to eat when you weren't hungry?
    no Did they encourage you to clean your plate? *no* Insist? *no*

24. Were you told you might get sick if you didn't eat at mealtime? *no*

25. When eating *at home* (and not dieting), which of the following do you usually
    eat at one meal? Salad ___✓___ Bread _____ Meat ___✓___ Vegetable ___✓___
    Dessert _____

26. When eating *out* (and not dieting), which of the following do you usually eat

32

at one meal? Salad _✓_ Bread _✓_ Meat _✓_ Vegetable _✓_
Dessert _✓_

27. Why do you believe you have a problem weighing what you want to weigh? *not disciplined enough to stay with it. Lifestyle includes many social events and dinners*

28. Why do you believe some people stay at normal weight without dieting? *They don't overeat.*

29. Is there anyone in your family or do you have a friend who is a True Thin (someone who is normal weight and never diets)? Indicate the relationship (son, mother, husband, daughter, etc.) *yes—friend*

30. Do you take any medication that we should know about? *take Corgard for high blood pressure*

31. Please make any additional comments about yourself or your lifestyle that you believe will enable us to help you in lowering your weight. *As mentioned above my wife and I go out socially a great deal—also we go to a great many banquets. We also travel a great deal and eat in nice restaurants in such places as New York, New Orleans, etc.*

YOUR EATING PROFILE

NAME _Sanford Reitman_   AGE _48_   HEIGHT _5'10"_

PRESENT WEIGHT _198_   GOAL WEIGHT _165_

1. When did your weight problem begin? (Time and/or event) _at birth_

2. List the last 4 diets you have tried, date, amount of weight lost, length of time.

Diet	Date	Amount Lost	Time on Diet
low calorie		_5_	_1 mo_
low carbo		_15_	_1 year_
low carbo		_64_	_9 months_
starvation		_7_	_1 week_

3. If you were overweight as a child, what years? _birth to 15 years_

4. What is the lowest you have weighed since age 23? _175_

5. On a normal weekend does your weight increase and, if so, how much? _1–3 lbs._

6. On a weekend trip does you weight increase and, if so, how much? _1–3 lbs._

7. Last year did you gain weight from Dec. 1 to Jan. 1? _yes_ How much? _6 lbs._ How long did it take to lower your weight back to your Dec. 1 weight? _1 month_

8. On the average, how much per year does your weight increase? *3 lbs.*

9. Is there a weight you cannot seem to go below no matter how hard you try? *yes* What is that weight? *175* When was the last time you weighed this? *age 24*

10. Which of the following do you eat regularly?

    _√_ Breakfast   ___ Mid-morning snack

    _√_ Lunch   ___ Mid-afternoon snack

    _√_ Dinner   _√_ After-dinner snack

11. If you usually eat breakfast, or a "little something," about what time? *6:30 a.m.* What do you eat and drink? *english muffin and butter, coffee*

12. How often do you eat cereal during the week? Daily ___ 5 × week ___

    3 × week ___ 1 × week ___ seldom/never _√_

13. Circle those of the following you usually drink: (JUICES) . . . COLD DRINKS (SUGARED) . . . MILK . . . HEALTH DRINKS . . . HOT/COLD CHOCOLATE . . . CUPS OF SOUP . . . MILK SHAKES

14. What are your favorite foods and snacks when you aren't dieting? *sandwiches*

15. What low calorie foods do you really enjoy? *all vegetables*

16. How often do you eat desserts? Daily ___ 5 × week ___ 3 × week ___

    1 × week ___ seldom/never _√_

17. Do you prefer soft or crunchy foods? *yes, yes* Both? ___ Spicy _√_ foods?

18. In order of preference, list kinds of bread you enjoy. *rye, whole wheat*

_____

19. Are you a SLOW or (FAST) eater? Circle one.

20. Do you leave food on your plate? Yes _____ No ✓
    How often? *never ever!*

21. Do you ordinarily take seconds? Yes ✓ No _____ If yes, is it because
    you ✓ are still hungry _____ usually do _____ urged to by parent,
    spouse, others

22. Do you eat more than usual or less when you are feeling:
    more depressed   *more* anxious
    " nervous   " excited
    " angry   " sad

23. As a child, did your parents encourage you to eat when you weren't hungry?
    yes Did they encourage you to clean your plate? *yes* Insist? *yes*

24. Were you told you might get sick if you didn't eat at mealtime? *no*

25. When eating *at home* (and not dieting), which of the following do you usually
    eat at one meal? Salad ✓ Bread _____ Meat ✓ Vegetable ✓
    Dessert _____

26. When eating *out* (and not dieting), which of the following do you usually eat
    at one meal? Salad ✓ Bread ✓ Meat ✓ Vegetable ✓
    Dessert _____

27. Why do you believe you have a problem weighing what you want to weigh?
    eating has become a hobby rather than a necessity

_____

28. Why do you believe some people stay at normal weight without dieting? *heredity, eating style, activity*

29. Is there anyone in your family or do you have a friend who is a True Thin (someone who is normal weight and never diets)? Indicate the relationship (son, mother, husband, daughter, etc.) *son, wife, daughter*

30. Do you take any medication that we should know about? *no*

31. Please make any additional comments about yourself or your lifestyle that you believe will enable us to help you in lowering your weight. *travel abroad frequently; entertain at home often; eat out often; gourmet cooking a hobby*

YOUR EATING PROFILE

NAME _Jack Wilson_   AGE _38_ HEIGHT _6'0"_

PRESENT WEIGHT _237½_   GOAL WEIGHT _180_

1. When did your weight problem begin? (Time and/or event) _early childhood_

2. List the last 4 diets you have tried, date, amount of weight lost, length of time.

Diet	Date	Amount Lost	Time on Diet
starvation	_79_	_35_	_2 months_

3. If you were overweight as a child, what years? _from 7 years on_

4. What is the lowest you have weighed since age 23? _200_

5. On a normal weekend does your weight increase and, if so, how much? _1 lb._

6. On a weekend trip does your weight increase and, if so, how much? _2 lbs._

7. Last year did you gain weight from Dec. 1 to Jan. 1? _yes_ How much? _1–2 lbs._ How long did it take to lower your weight back to your Dec. 1 weight? _never_

8. On the average, how much per year does your weight increase? *5–8 lbs.*

9. Is there a weight you cannot seem to go below no matter how hard you try? *no* What is that weight? _____ When was the last time you weighed this?

10. Which of the following do you eat regularly?

    Breakfast _____   Mid-morning snack _____

    Lunch _✓_   Mid-afternoon snack _____

    Dinner _✓_   After-dinner snack _✓_

11. If you usually eat breakfast, or a "little something," about what time? *6:30* *a.m.* What do you eat and drink? *cereal*

12. How often do you eat cereal during the week? Daily _____ 5 × week _____ 3 × week _____ 1 × week _✓_ seldom/never _____

13. Circle those of the following you usually drink: (JUICES) . . (COLD DRINKS (SUGARED)) . . (MILK) . . HEALTH DRINKS . . . HOT/COLD CHOCOLATE . . . CUPS OF SOUP . . . MILK SHAKES

14. What are your favorite foods and snacks when you aren't dieting? *ice cream, peanut butter, cookies, candy, all fattening things*

15. What low calorie foods do you really enjoy? *almost all vegetables, fish, chicken, salad, diet Dr. Pepper*

16. How often do you eat desserts? Daily _✓_ 5 × week _____ 3 × week _____ 1 × week _____ seldom/never _____

17. Do you prefer soft or crunchy foods? *soft* Both? _____ Spicy foods? *yes*

39

18. In order of preference, list kinds of bread you enjoy. *almost any bread with butter*

19. Are you a SLOW or (FAST) eater? Circle one.

20. Do you leave food on your plate? Yes _____ No √
    How often? _____

21. Do you ordinarily take seconds? Yes _____ No √   If yes, is it because
    you _____ are still hungry √   usually do _____   urged to by parent,
    spouse, others _____

22. Do you eat more than usual or less when you are feeling:
    more depressed   *more* anxious
    " nervous   " excited
    " angry   " sad

23. As a child, did your parents encourage you to eat when you weren't hungry?
    no Did they encourage you to clean your plate? *yes* Insist? *no*

24. Were you told you might get sick if you didn't eat at mealtime? *no*

25. When eating *at home* (and not dieting), which of the following do you usually
    eat at one meal? Salad √ Bread √ Meat √ Vegetable √
    Dessert √

26. When eating *out* (and not dieting), which of the following do you usually eat
    at one meal? Salad √ Bread √ Meat √ Vegetable √
    Dessert √

27. Why do you believe you have a problem weighing what you want to weigh?
    I eat so fast I still feel hungry so I always eat second helping

40

28. Why do you believe some people stay at normal weight without dieting? *Eat right foods, eat slower*

29. Is there anyone in your family or do you have a friend who is a True Thin (someone who is normal weight and never diets)? Indicate the relationship (son, mother, husband, daughter, etc.) *wife*

30. Do you take any medication that we should know about? *no*

31. Please make any additional comments about yourself or your lifestyle that you believe will enable us to help you in lowering your weight. *I want to lose weight and I want to keep it off*

YOUR EATING PROFILE

NAME _____ AGE _____ HEIGHT _____

PRESENT WEIGHT _____ GOAL WEIGHT _____

1. When did your weight problem begin? (Time and/or event)
   _____

2. List the last 4 diets you have tried, date, amount of weight lost, length of time.

Diet	Date	Amount Lost	Time on Diet
_____	_____	_____	_____
_____	_____	_____	_____
_____	_____	_____	_____
_____	_____	_____	_____

3. If you were overweight as a child, what years? _____

4. What is the lowest you have weighed since age 23? _____

5. On a normal weekend does your weight increase and, if so, how much? _____

6. On a weekend trip does your weight increase and, if so, how much? _____

7. Last year did you gain weight from Dec. 1 to Jan. 1? _____ How much? _____ How long did it take to lower your weight back to your Dec. 1 weight? _____

42

8. On the average, how much per year does your weight increase? _____

9. Is there a weight you cannot seem to go below no matter how hard you try? _____ What is that weight? _____ When was the last time you weighed this? _____

10. Which of the following do you eat regularly?
   _____ Breakfast   _____ Mid-morning snack
   _____ Lunch   _____ Mid-afternoon snack
   _____ Dinner   _____ After-dinner snack

11. If you usually eat breakfast, or a "little something," about what time? _____ What do you eat and drink? _____
   _____

12. How often do you eat cereal during the week? Daily _____ 5 × week _____ 3 × week _____ 1 × week _____ seldom/never _____

13. Circle those of the following you usually drink: JUICES . . . COLD DRINKS (SUGARED) . . . MILK . . . HEALTH DRINKS . . . HOT/COLD CHOCOLATE . . . CUPS OF SOUP . . . MILK SHAKES

14. What are your favorite foods and snacks when you aren't dieting? _____
   _____

15. What low calorie foods do you really enjoy? _____
   _____

16. How often do you eat desserts? Daily _____ 5 × week _____ 3 × week _____ 1 × week _____ seldom/never _____

17. Do you prefer soft or crunchy foods? _____ Both? _____ Spicy foods? _____

18. In order of preference, list kinds of bread you enjoy. _____

19. Are you a SLOW or FAST eater? Circle one.

20. Do you leave food on your plate? Yes _____ No _____
    How often? _____

21. Do you ordinarily take seconds? Yes _____ No _____ If yes, is it because
    you _____ are still hungry _____ usually do _____ urged to by parent,
    spouse, others _____

22. Do you eat more than usual or less when you are feeling:
    _____ depressed
    _____ nervous
    _____ angry
    _____ anxious
    _____ excited
    _____ sad

23. As a child, did your parents encourage you to eat when you weren't hungry?
    _____ Did they encourage you to clean your plate? _____ Insist? _____

24. Were you told you might get sick if you didn't eat at mealtime? _____

25. When eating *at home* (and not dieting), which of the following do you usually
    eat at one meal? Salad _____ Bread _____ Meat _____ Vegetable _____
    Dessert _____

26. When eating *out* (and not dieting), which of the following do you usually eat
    at one meal? Salad _____ Bread _____ Meat _____ Vegetable _____
    Dessert _____

27. Why do you believe you have a problem weighing what you want to weigh?
    _____

44

28. Why do you believe some people stay at normal weight without dieting?

_____

29. Is there anyone in your family or do you have a friend who is a True Thin (someone who is normal weight and never diets)? Indicate the relationship (son, mother, husband, daughter, etc.)

_____

30. Do you take any medication that we should know about?

_____

31. Please make any additional comments about yourself or your lifestyle that you believe will enable us to help you in lowering your weight.

_____

_____

_____

DR. WAYNE AGNEW'S CAPSULE COMMENTS:

The YOUR EATING PROFILE forms you have just looked at in this chapter gave Sandra Breithaupt and me quite a bit of useful information on Doctors Bane, Daniel, Mendelson, Pirtle, Reitman and Wilson's eating habits and attitudes toward food. Every doctor eats too fast. Every doctor reaches for food when under emotional and physical stress. Every one of the doctors has been fighting the problem of regaining or maintaining a normal weight.

The eating profiles give even more clues to the causes of the doctors' weight problems:

Dr. Jerry Bane is a heavy milk drinker, a daily dessert eater, and a believer that every dinner should include salad, bread, meat, vegetables and dessert. He also feels he has to clean his plate, a pattern left over from his childhood. On the good side, Dr. Bane is not a snacker or weekend binger and he is realistic in his weight-loss goal of 21 pounds, as he has weighed this amount before as an adult.

Dr. Cliff Daniel doesn't list *any* goal weight, which indicates he is open to a weight loss he can feel comfortable with, instead of fantasizing about trying to get back to his all-time bottom weight of 160 pounds, which is too low for his height. Although Dr. Daniel states that he likes crunchy foods, he is a heavy dessert, cereal and bread eater, and drinks many protein milk shakes, none of which give him any chewing satisfaction. Dr. Daniel was told in childhood that he would get sick if he didn't eat at mealtime, which helps explain why he eats to make himself feel better when under stress—he's still eating to stay well. You will note that his answer on Question 27 shows that he has trouble distinguishing hunger from feelings. And he *thinks* he craves desserts, but notice his answers to Questions 25 and 26: he always eats desserts when at home, but not when he dines out. If he wasn't served desserts, most of the time he probably wouldn't miss them.

Dr. Michael Mendelson's weight problem began after he entered medical practice. He has gained 54 pounds in the last ten years. A major reason for this increase is that he drinks his food instead of eating it, living on hot chocolate, sugary cold drinks and fruit juices all day long. Since he doesn't ordinarily eat breakfast or lunch, he probably believes that since he has skipped these meals he has a right to make it up at dinner and therefore overeats at his one real meal. Also, Dr. Mendelson doesn't eat foods he really loves; he says he appreciates food, yet he isn't aware enough of his food tastes to be able to list even one food that is important to him. He appears to look for what he can eat fast rather than what he actually enjoys.

Dr. Bill Pirtle is an old hand at dieting, especially deprivation diets. This accounts for the fact that when he eats out he eats everything—salad, bread, meat, vegetables, dessert. He feels he is temporarily out of diet prison and therefore eats everything he can get his fork into while he is free from restraints. Notice that he gains weight on weekends and over holidays. He obviously starts back on his diet on Monday, because at home he eats only salad, meat and vegetables. Dr. Pirtle is also confused about his true food preferences. He comments that he doesn't care that much for spicy foods (Question 17), but then lists the highly spicy Mexican foods as his favorites. He also faces the problem of being tempted by many exciting, rich foods, as his lifestyle includes numerous social events, travel and dinners in fine restaurants.

Dr. Sanford Reitman was overweight from early childhood until age fifteen, thanks to his parents' placing great importance on his cleaning his plate and eating to feel better.

His goal weight of 165 is a bit unrealistic for a person whose hobby is cooking and eating. Like Dr. Pirtle, he is locked into the "binge on weekends/diet on weekdays" syndrome, and he also is a deprivation dieter. Dr. Reitman blames his weight problem on heredity, not realizing that if he adapted his eating style to that of his True Thin wife, son and daughter, his "hereditary" problem would disappear along with his excess weight. He will learn how to accomplish this in succeeding chapters.

Dr. Jack Wilson drinks his food—juices, carbonated soft drinks and milk—and probably does not count such liquids as eating. He complicates this problem by preferring soft foods, which disappear down the throat quickly, since they don't need much chewing; and he eats very fast, which means that he has to take second helpings because he still feels hungry. Dr. Wilson believes all the foods he *likes* are fattening and that people who don't have weight problems don't eat these delicious foods, only "the right," low-calorie foods. Most people obese from childhood think this. He will learn on the Dallas Doctors' Diet program that he won't have to subsist on low-calorie foods to get thin.

My own eating profile revealed to me that like Doctors Pirtle and Reitman, I was a weekend/holiday binger and a weekday dieter, and also a deprivation dieter. I also drank a lot of my food in the forms of juices, milk, health drinks and soup, ate around feelings, always cleaned my plate, ordinarily took second helpings and *was convinced that my life-long obesity was due to eating too much.* This is only partially true, and you will learn WHY in this book!

2

FOOD
IS NOT
YOUR PROBLEM

TEACHING A GROUP of conservative doctors how to lose weight was going to be one of the major challenges of my life, I realized, as I looked around the room at the faces of the Dallas doctors Dr. Wayne Agnew had gathered together.

The doctors were polite but clearly dubious that I, a woman with no medical training, could help them solve their own personal obesity problems.

Wayne gave me an encouraging smile. Praying that my nervousness didn't show, I began to talk: "Welcome to Naturally Slim. I feel that our program is very exciting and I'm very honored to be able to present it to you. What I am going to describe to you tonight is a revolutionary new way of eating that is based on age-old good sense, good health and knowing your particular biochemical individuality.

"I know you have all tried other diets in the past. A number of those, I'm sure you will agree with me, were nutritionally unsound, awkward to stay on when out socially, freaky in concept and practice, and, worst of all, were *deprivation* diets. The Naturally Slim program has none of these drawbacks. You will be able to eat most of the foods you really crave—those favorite foods of yours—in reasonable quantities every day, and you will burn off fat while doing so *if* you eat *only* when I tell you to. For you see, *food is not your problem; WHEN you eat is.*

"Primitive man ate only when he was hungry and so never had a weight problem. Modern man eats not when his body tells him to, but when civilization tells him to. This is called Clock Dictated Eating, and in this program you will learn how to change your fat-producing 'civilized' cycle for your innate skinny, 'primitive' pattern.

"You will also learn the difference between satiety and fullness so that you will never be subject to destructive food binges again . . .

"and how separating appetite from hunger will make the pounds melt off of you and even keep you from suffering through those frustrating plateaus that are an unhappy part of other diets . . .

"plus you will find out that one of the 'primitive' keys to melting those pounds off you will be water—not used to turn you into a walking swimming pool, like the Stillman diet did, but to increase intracellular Fat-Burn-Out action."

I could see looks of puzzlement on the doctors' faces.

"I am an unvarying size four and I stay that way by eating only the 'bad' foods I love instead of the wilted spinach and celery diets I lived on while I was hopelessly obese.

"Tonight for dinner I had a stuffed artichoke swimming in butter, lobster with crabmeat stuffing, a baked potato drenched with more butter and sour cream, tossed salad with blue cheese dressing, eight small pieces of garlic toast and two glasses of water . . . and I will not gain a single, solitary pound from this feast of supposedly fattening foods."

The doctors looked at me as if I was touched in the head.

"I eat dinners like this as often as I please and never gain weight, but nine years ago when I was nibbling away at carrot sticks, grapefruit and skinned chicken breasts I was just like you when you diet—hungry, irritable, ashamed, and never able to quite attain, much less stay at, my ideal weight.

"I envied and almost hated those True Thins who could eat anything and not gain an ounce. I felt anger and bitterness at having been fated to be a permanent overweight even though I had done nothing to deserve it.

"I was always yo-yoing—punishing myself with each season's new wonder diet long enough to become thin and then rewarding myself for having been in 'diet prison' by breaking loose and binging on all my favorite foods, such as crabmeat Jambalaya, quiche Lorraine and mounds of chicken salad with *real* mayonnaise.

"Does this sound familiar? Do you feel, after years of failing to become thin despite trying each season's new 'guaranteed' diet, that only a miracle can save you from living the rest of your lives encased in ever-thickening amounts of jiggly fat? Well, by learning to eat only when hungry, you will activate your Fat-Burn-Out mechanism and become a normal True Thin person again. You see, what I didn't realize most of my life was that the reason I was obese was not because of *what* I ate, but *how* I ate. On the Naturally Slim program you truly don't have to count calories. You will be able to eat nearly all of the really fattening foods such as bread, rolls, pasta, cheeses and sauces, and you will *lose*, not gain weight."

Dr. Sandy Reitman was objecting. "The basic logic of obesity is that you're always eating more than you need to sustain yourself. The secret to losing weight is to take in *less* than you need for a while. You can't eat rolls, pasta and sauces every day and expect to lose weight."

Dr. Bill Pirtle agreed. "You have so many people who come into their doctor and say, 'I've gained twenty pounds in the last two months and I just don't eat anything, Doctor.' They're kidding themselves. Calories do count. They've been eating too much."

"I myself see many patients," said Dr. Mike Mendelson, "who have had problems being overweight. I kinda tell them they have a problem with *calories*. The classic story is, the patient says, 'I don't know why I'm so fat. I'm eating like a feather, hardly *anything*. Why do you think that is?' And I tell them. The classic thing you tell them is that in the concentration camps in Germany they had all kinds—they had 'em thin and they had 'em fat, they had pituitary disease and thyroid disease and diabetes and hypertension, the whole gamut—but the one thing they weren't when they left those concentration camps was *fat*. And the reason for that was, they weren't getting enough calories. When you're eating grass or wood or mattress, you aren't putting any calories on. You get very skinny. I ask them, 'You ever see any people from there?'

"They say, 'Well, yeah . . .'

"The problem is that the calories you're taking in are more than the body needs. So one has to correct that problem. If you're hypothyroid, you're not efficiently getting rid of your energy stores, but that's okay—if you take in less, you'll lose weight. You have to take in less to lose weight."

Oh, dear. We were only a few minutes into the first session and already I had a mutiny on my hands! But I continued.

"I understand why you are questioning what I'm saying, but remember, Doctor Agnew is as sensible and cautious and knowledgeable a medical man as you are, and he has come to believe that the principles of Naturally Slim are healthy, sound and practical. He is living proof that you don't have to count calories, that you can eat your favorite foods and actually lose weight. Wayne, how much have you lost so far?"

"Thirty-two pounds."

"Could you name a few of your favorite foods that you have continued to eat while on the Naturally Slim diet?"

"Well, Wanda's chicken enchiladas, which are superb; chalupas; tacos; steak and potatoes."

I turned back to the Dallas doctors. "I want you to forget," I said firmly, "everything you know about dieting. Just clear all your previous conceptions out of your head, for nothing you know now will apply to *your* weight problem. After all, if calorie counting, high-protein/low-carbohydrate, fasting, enzymes, high-grain diets and the like had worked for you, you wouldn't be sitting here now still overweight.

"The first step in understanding my diet is to learn the difference between True Thins and Overeaters.

"True Thins are people who never have a weight problem and yet eat anything they want to, *when* they want to. They pay no attention to calories. In fact, if you told them they shouldn't eat something because it is fattening and contains too many calories, they would just look at you quizzically and then return to eating the 'bad' food. And, of course, the True Thin is right, for eating 'bad' or non-diet foods doesn't put weight on the True Thin. All it does is make them enjoy their meal that much more since they are eating something really delicious that they hunger for.

"The Overeaters, on the other hand, live in the world of 'good' and 'bad' foods. There are the good foods they hate but eat anyway because this will keep their weight from skyrocketing; and the 'bad' foods they love but never allow themselves the pleasure of having except during periodic, guilt-ridden eating binges. During these binges, I might add, the Overeater usually regains all the weight he or she took off and maintained on his or her 'good' regimen, plus a few more pounds for good measure. So the Overeater is usually prey to the yo-yo syndrome: fat/thin, fat/thin, fat again, which puts his or her body under great stress and is therefore a medically unsound way of life.

"What you, the Overeater, don't realize, however, is that you've *become* an Overeater. You were born a True Thin and can become one again *by learning to eat only when you are hungry.*

"This DIALOGUE CHART will show you when, what, how and why the Overeater (that's you *now*) and the True Thin (you to *be*) eat" (Figure 1).

DIALOGUE BETWEEN THE

OVEREATER AND TRUE THIN

About When to Eat

OVEREATER: "Even though I'm not hungry in the morning, I always eat breakfast."

TRUE THIN: *"Why? Are you really hungry when you first get up? I'm not, so I don't eat breakfast."*

OVEREATER: "No, I've never been hungry then, but it's important to start the day with something in your stomach."

TRUE THIN: *"I wait until I feel hungry to eat something. That's usually around 10:30 a.m."*

OVEREATER: "Don't you feel odd eating breakfast food at 10:30?"

TRUE THIN: *"I don't eat breakfast food then or any other time because I've never liked breakfast food."*

What to Eat

OVEREATER: "What do you eat then?"

TRUE THIN: *"It depends. Sometimes I have crackers and cheese, or open a can of sardines, or even have some ice cream."*

OVEREATER: "Ice cream! I only allow myself to eat ice cream when I'm on a food binge. Normally, I'm very careful and restrict myself to low-calorie foods at breakfast, lunch and dinner."

55

TRUE THIN: *"I, unfortunately, am not usually hungry when the clock says I should be. . . ."*

OVEREATER: "I'm always hungry."

TRUE THIN: *"I'm only hungry about twice a day—at 10:30 and around 4 or 5 in late afternoon. So that's when I eat."*

How Much to Eat

OVEREATER: "But I don't understand how you stay so thin eating those fattening foods you just mentioned."

TRUE THIN: *"I don't know."* (shrug) *"And when I do eat, people call me the human vacuum cleaner."*

OVEREATER: "Have you ever had a weight problem?"

TRUE THIN: *"No, but occasionally I do get five pounds heavier than I'd like, so I just stop eating sweets and eat less for a week or so. I lose the excess weight with no problem."*

Current Weight

OVEREATER: "What do you weigh now?"

TRUE THIN: *"I don't know. I don't own a scale."*

OVEREATER: "I'm always fat and I seem to live on scales."

TRUE THIN: *"I know when I'm gaining because my clothes get tighter."*

OVEREATER: "When I'm gaining, I just move into my next larger size set of clothes. I have my thin clothes, my plump clothes, and my disgustingly fat clothes."

What Special Foods Represent

TRUE THIN: *"What do you do when you food binge? I'm just curious."*

OVEREATER: "I eat all the delicious things that I crave the rest of the time but don't allow myself to have—things like chocolate chip cookies made with pure butter, fettucini Alfredo, and my favorite, banana cream pie."

TRUE THIN: *"I love banana cream pie too. Sometimes I just skip dinner entirely and get right to the main course—a banana cream pie."*

OVEREATER: "My mother makes the world's best banana cream pie. It's loaded with bananas and piled high with real whipped cream. I dream about it sometimes."

Feelings about Food

TRUE THIN: *"You dream about food!"*

OVEREATER: "I dream about it, I think about it, I talk about it with my other fat friends, I subscribe to gourmet magazines just so I can feast on the pictures, and I read about it in my enormous collection of cookbooks. Food is *very* important to me."

"The messages in this chart will become crystal clear to you in the next three weeks. For now, all you have to understand is that by learning the when, what, how principles of the True Thin you can expect to lose two to ten pounds the first week, and two to three pounds each succeeding week without ever feeling hungry or eating less than you want to of your favorite foods . . . except for the first two weeks when you aren't allowed to have any fruit juices, commercial dry cereals, milk or sweets. Anything else goes, including a drink before dinner if you wish. Furthermore, during Week Three of my diet, you will be able to add back in your favorite sweets such as banana cream pie, ice cream and even candy, and *still* continue to lose weight. I know you think these are impossible promises for me to keep, but you will feel differently after a few days on this diet program.

"I am truly excited about helping you to become thin again. Losing weight cannot and should not be drudgery! I know that if you and I work with your body we will get you slim and keep you that way. I have done most of the work for you. The principles and guidelines I am passing on to you took over five years and three thousand overweight people made skinny again to perfect, so all you have to do is follow my instructions exactly on how to happily eat your way thin and you *will* become thin and stay that way for the rest of your life!

"Lesson number one will be how to identify your own highly individual hunger pattern."

DR. WAYNE AGNEW'S CAPSULE COMMENTS:

On Sandra Breithaupt's Naturally Slim diet you will learn how to change yourself from an Overeater into a True Thin.

1. You will avoid the diet foods you hate and feast on most of your favorite, supposedly fattening foods.
2. Your weight loss of 2 to 10 pounds in the first week and 2 to 3 pounds each succeeding week will be accomplished because you will be eating only when you are really hungry.
3. This new way of eating is the healthiest, easiest-to-

maintain diet program I have ever experienced, but I strongly recommend that before you start this or any other diet you seek the advice and consent of your own physician to make sure that you don't have a medical condition that would preclude your going on a weight-loss program at this time.

3

YOUR HUNGER PATTERN: THE KEY TO PERMANENT WEIGHT LOSS

EVERY OVERWEIGHT PERSON knows what appetite is . . . a wish or craving for foods that are highly desirable to you. Chocolate chip cookies perhaps, or fresh raspberries or newly baked bread.

Appetite can be triggered by sight, smell, memory or anticipation.

Hunger cannot.

Hunger is the physical need of the body for food to keep your physiological processes working. Your stomach does not care what you fill it with—a cheeseburger or lettuce and carrots—the stomach has no taste buds or emotional needs; it only knows when it is comfortable and when it is *empty*.

Hunger is the body's physical signal that it *needs* food, any food, to sustain life.

Appetite, on the other hand, is the intellectual, emotional and sensuous longing for specific foods to enhance pleasure.

Fat people know a lot about appetite, but when hunger is defined for them as above, they would be hard put to remember the last time they actually experienced hunger.

And that is why they are fat.

If you are obese it is because you don't know the difference between appetite and hunger and therefore eat before your body is ready and able efficiently to utilize the food you are giving it.

At the beginning of this book I told you that it was something that a True Thin said in passing that made me realize why I was different from the naturally slim people of this world. It wasn't my "glands," or that I was born with fat cells, or that I ingested more food than thin people. No, I was overweight because I didn't know WHEN to eat. What the True Thin man said that night was, "I only eat when I'm hungry." Give this deceptively simple statement your closest attention, for it can change your life.

WHEN you eat will determine whether you stay fat or become thin, not WHAT you eat.

Why? Let's go back and take another look at our ancestors. To survive, early man had to be highly sensitive to his body's needs, and so primitive man taught himself to identify hunger and thirst signals and act upon them. When your ancestor's body needed more fuel, it told him so and then, *and only then,* man ate. He didn't nibble or snack. He didn't gnaw on a carcass just because the

Neanderthal in the next cave was eating. Primitive man was never conditioned by the society he lived in to distort the naturally efficient fuel intake pattern of his body, so he never became fat.

Modern man won't become fat either, if he eats (1) only when hungry and (2) only until full.

It's that simple. The True Thin eats only when hungry, so he doesn't burden his or her body with food it can't efficiently utilize.

Overeaters stuff their bodies with food when appetite lures them into eating. Therefore they clog up their bodies with excess food that their systems can't burn up (Fat-Burn-Out) or get rid of, so the system does the next best thing—stores it as fat.

Have you ever tried to stuff more coal into a full furnace? The fire was partially smothered, burned the coal more slowly, and gave off *less* heat, right? But when you waited until the fire was running low to shovel in more coal, the furnace put out plenty of heat. If you wait until supplies are low to shovel in the pizza or roast duck or two-foot submarine sandwich, your body won't have any fat left over to store on your waist, hips and thighs, because your body, needing your fuel, will burn everything you eat right up. Fat-Burn-Out will take place.

You are going to have to learn the difference between hunger and appetite signals and act only upon the former to achieve daily Fat-Burn-Out. My research has shown me that people potentially go through four stages of hunger levels:

LEVEL 1—No hunger
LEVEL 2—Appetite

LEVEL 3—True hunger
LEVEL 4—Overhunger

At HUNGER LEVEL 1, you don't feel any desire for food. At HUNGER LEVEL 2, your appetite has been stirred, perhaps by the sight of a TV commercial or by smelling something delicious cooking, or remembering something wonderful you've eaten before or because you're anticipating a particular treat . . . maybe the luncheon special today at the restaurant you patronize is going to be your favorite version of chicken and dumplings, and even though you're not hungry, your taste buds are setting up a clamor for this delicacy. HUNGER LEVEL 3 is the point where you actually feel and are hungry. This is the magic period when anything you eat will be assimilated by the body because all your hormones, enzymes and cellular action are at peak efficiency, allowing Fat-Burn-Out to take place. HUNGER LEVEL 4 is a stage few Overeaters are familiar with: this is when you've become *too* hungry . . . ravenous . . . to be able to control your food intake; you snatch and swallow almost anything you can get your hands on and mouth around.

My HUNGER LEVEL COMPUTER should help you become aware of when you're actually hungry (LEVEL 3) or just responding to the siren song of appetite.

HUNGER LEVEL COMPUTER

LEVEL 1—NO HUNGER

Seeing, smelling or thinking about food doesn't provoke any desire in you to eat.

LEVEL 2—APPETITE

The idea of certain favorite foods is tantalizing. At LEVEL 2 you would be tempted to eat a few potato chips or cookies or canapes if they were placed before you, but you wouldn't be "hungry for" a green salad without dressing or a leftover hamburger casserole if it was offered to you.

LEVEL 2 is the stage when you are likely to wander out to the kitchen and look in the refrigerator to see if anything there "interests" you. *But if you don't know what you want to eat, then you're not hungry.*

At LEVEL 2 appetite can seduce you into wanting to eat something, *even if you are full,* but obviously, *if you are full, you can't be hungry!*

OVEREATERS REACH HUNGER LEVEL 2 MANY TIMES DURING THE DAY AND EVENING.

LEVEL 3—TRUE HUNGER

At this point even lettuce leaves and leftover casseroles begin to look good to you. Your body is giving out strong "I'm empty" signals to you (some peoples' stomachs even emit rumbling sounds at LEVEL 3), you are aware of a healthy, pleasurable urge to fill up and will tackle your food with zest and eat until comfortably full.

YOU WILL REACH LEVEL 3 ONE TO THREE TIMES EACH DAY.

LEVEL 4—OVERHUNGER

This level is as dangerous to your attempts to lose

weight as LEVEL 2, for at LEVEL 4, when you are too hungry, you will eat anything in sight, gobble it down without pleasure and eat past the point of satiety.

Some physical signs or symptoms of LEVEL 4 may be weakness, nausea or headache.

Some emotional symptoms may be inability to concentrate, irritability or depression.

LEVEL 4 usually occurs forty minutes to two hours after you reach LEVEL 3, if you don't eat then.

It is crucial that you learn to identify when you are at HUNGER LEVEL 3, for that is the only time you can safely eat and not gain weight. When you are at LEVEL 3 you can eat any and all foods you please (with the exceptions of fruit and vegetable juices, cereals, milk and, for the first two weeks, sweets) until you are full, but during the rest of the time you are not allowed to have so much as an orange or a cracker, for ANY FOODS EATEN WHEN YOU ARE NOT HUNGRY WILL SABOTAGE YOUR FAT-BURN-OUT MECHANISM AND CAUSE YOU TO *GAIN*, NOT LOSE WEIGHT!

Identifying when you are hungry will at first be confusing to you. Overeaters nearly always tell me, "Sandra, I'm *always* hungry." But that's not so. During my years of teaching my Naturally Slim courses I have discovered that 65% of us get hungry only *twice* a day (two-time-a-day hunger), 15% get hungry *once* a day (one-time-a-day hunger), and 5% of us get hungry *three* times a day (three-time-a-day hunger). The other 15% of us have two-time-a-day hunger some days and one-time-a-day hunger other days, depending upon the amount we eat and the richness of the food.

You are probably going to fall into that 65% category, which means that if you have been eating more than twice a day, even if that food is diet food, you have been sabotaging your Fat-Burn-Out mechanism. Wouldn't you rather eat less often, if when you do eat you can have all you want of your favorite foods and lose weight in the process? If so, you are ready to follow my instructions for Week One of my Naturally Slim course.

DR. WAYNE AGNEW'S CAPSULE COMMENTS:

It's ironic that as mature individuals we have to relearn something we already knew as babies—to eat only when hungry. If you will observe babies at around five or six months when they are just beginning to eat actual foods, you will notice that they indicate they want food by opening their mouths and leaning forward, and they show they are full by leaning back and turning their heads away. So even before we can talk, we are able to tell when we have reached HUNGER LEVEL 3, and when we are comfortably full. Therefore we certainly can figure out how to tell the difference between appetite and hunger now that we are adults.

Your first step in shedding weight will be to use the HUNGER LEVEL COMPUTER to identify the four stages of hunger—no hunger, appetite, true hunger, overhunger. This information will enable you to determine whether you have

- three-time-a-day hunger
- two-time-a-day hunger
- one-time-a-day hunger
- two-time-a-day hunger some days and one-time-a-day hunger other days.

4

WEEK ONE OF THE DALLAS DOCTORS' DIET

STEP ONE

Eat Only When at HUNGER LEVEL 3

YOUR FIRST ASSIGNMENT is to discover your individual hunger pattern . . . the one that is unique to your body. To do that, I am going to ask you NOT TO EAT BREAKFAST FOR THE FIRST THREE DAYS, EVEN IF YOU THINK YOU ARE HUNGRY FIRST THING IN THE MORNING.

Why am I making this odd request? Because this is the only way you will discover if you are a "morning hunger" individual.

You may have up to three cups of coffee or tea (with a *conservative* amount of sugar and cream) if you feel you can't start the day without your usual caffeine fix,

67

but YOU ARE NOT TO TAKE ONE BITE OF FOOD FOR THE FIRST THREE DAYS UNTIL YOU ARE SURE YOU HAVE REACHED HUNGER LEVEL 3. This may be at any time . . . 10:30 . . . 11:00 . . . 12:00 . . . or even afternoon.

When you do reach HUNGER LEVEL 3, eat until you are full and then don't touch any food again until you are *positive* that you are hungry.

If you find yourself baffled about whether you are at HUNGER LEVEL 2 or HUNGER LEVEL 3, it may be that you are one of the many people who confuse hunger with thirst. Drink a glass of water and wait fifteen minutes. If you still feel hungry, you probably are (more about water drinking later).

You are going to find yourself eating at some odd times, but don't let that bother you. Your body will soon thank you for restoring it to its normal food intake cycle, and you will have the added incentives of being able to eat foods that are highly pleasurable to you and at the same time seeing the pointer on your bathroom scales creeping backward.

Next, write down the time of day you eat each meal and what you ate on your Food Sheet. (Instructions for filling out these sheets will be given to you at the end of this chapter.)

Be prepared to feel uncomfortable, even guilty about skipping breakfast this first three days. Actually, you won't be skipping any meals. When you are not eating, your body will be. It will be eating your fat!

We have been brainwashed for most of our lives to believe that if we don't "start the day with a little something in our stomachs" we won't be able to function well, and indeed, for 5% of the population, this is so. But for most of us, eating breakfast when we're not hungry will make us falsely hungry all day long. This is doubly bad, for false hunger is much more uncomfortable and uncontrollable than true hunger. It keeps you insatiable, craving food continuously throughout the day and into the night. As one Shreveport real-estate executive who has to take clients to luscious lunches and then fix food for her family in the evening said, "All these years I have been eating a poached egg on toast each morning to keep my strength up, when all I have accomplished was to turn on my 'hunger motor' and make myself ravenous for lunch and starving for dinner." She lost 14 pounds in three weeks when she stopped eating the egg and toast at HUNGER LEVEL 1 when her body wasn't hungry.

What is the history of breakfast? We are the descendants of an agricultural society. Our ancestors worked farms and plantations or else they worked their own piece of land for their food. The pattern of these people was that they generally started their day about 4:00 A.M. The cows were milked, field workers entered the fields, the women started building fires and readying the kitchen for the morning meal to be served about 7:00 or 8:00 A.M. These people ate breakfast *after* putting in three or four hours of hard work! They were definitely hungry. Most people have no need for food when they arise. The most work they do in the morning before leaving the house is dressing! The housewife doesn't have to eat either . . . she hasn't done any work yet.

Nor do you have to eat breakfast while you practically have one foot still in bed.

STEP TWO

Eat Anything You Want, but Taste Your Food

There are 10,000 taste buds in your mouth just sitting

there waiting for you to turn them on. True Thins give their taste buds a real workout with every bite they take, but Overeaters have deprived taste buds. Why? Because Overeaters take big bites and swallow those bites before their taste buds have a chance to become fully activated. If you will take this little food test with me you will see what I mean. Assemble a "taster plate" of four potato chips, six peanuts and one-half ounce of cheese.

Potato Chips. You are probably used to eating a large bag of potato chips at one sitting, but now you are going to eat four potato chips and be satisfied. Potato chips are a food that you eat when you are off your diet, therefore they are usually gobbled. You do this because you think you should not be eating them, right? You feel you have to hurry up and polish them off to get rid of the evidence of the crime, so to speak.

Now I want you to pick up the first chip and smell it. What kind is it? Barbecue? Onion? Garlic? Cheese? Is this the first time you've noticed that potato chips have a smell? How could we enjoy food if we didn't have that wonderful sense of smell?

Place the chip on your tongue, but don't bite down. Now pull it away. Did you taste the salt? Stop and realize that you have not eaten this food yet. Rarely do Overeaters hold a food very long in their hands before eating it. How do you feel knowing that you haven't eaten this potato chip yet?

Chew the chip and enjoy it. Take bites of it. Don't put the whole chip in your mouth at once, just enjoy it. You are going to be able to lose weight eating potato chips, and you want to learn how many it will take to satisfy you.

Take another potato chip. Take a bite, a big bite. Don't chew it, just let it m-e-l-t. You know, grownups never let food melt in their mouths. Children do. They do it all the time when they are small and we *wrongly* fuss at them, telling them "Don't hold food in your mouth! Chew it up and swallow it!" Well I want you to eat this potato chip as you would have when you were six years old. Notice how you really taste that chip when you let it melt in your mouth?

Go ahead now and finish this chip, chewing it slowly and enjoying it.

Take your next potato chip and chew it up as fast as you can! Does it feel more like your daily way of eating to chew something up fast and swallow it in one big glump? The goal of the Overeater always seems to be swallowing, never chewing and tasting. The mouth of fat people is often only a subway station that food passes through on its fast way to the stomach! You're going to learn that slowing down has a great reward—taste.

Now take that last potato chip and really enjoy it. Move it around in your mouth . . . side to side . . . top to bottom. Savor its saltiness, texture, flavor, crunchiness.

After you have eaten four potato chips ask yourself if you really feel as if you have enjoyed potato chips more eating them slowly instead of popping several at a time in your mouth. Do you *like* potato chips now that you have tasted them, or do you prefer corn chips or no chips at all? Are you beginning to think more about the kinds of tastes, smells and textures that give you pleasure? When we can eat all foods freely, then we become more discerning about our own individual appetite for certain foods.

Peanuts. Pick up one of your peanuts. You may feel funny picking up just one, when you have undoubtedly become accustomed to picking up a whole handful and stuffing them into your mouth at once, but I want you to start with one peanut. Smell it. What kind is it? When you become sensitive to food you will notice that each brand smells different. Planter's, for example, has a very distinctive smell that you should be able to identify from all others.

Put the one nut in your mouth and let it melt. What is the flavor like? Salty again? Chew it up slowly.

Put another nut in your mouth. Don't chew it, but use your teeth to break the nut in half, then let the coating melt off. Now chew. What was that like?

Put another nut in and slowly chew it up, moving it around in your mouth the whole while. Be sure to let your whole mouth experience the food, not just your teeth. They are just for chewing. It is your mouth that is built for *tasting*. It is your mouth that is going to make your satiety center register.

Pick up your next nut and *throw* it into your mouth. Chew it up as fast as you can. Did it feel like salty air?

Now finish the last two nuts. Let them melt and then chew.

How do you feel eating only six peanuts? Most people say, "I feel I can taste *one* nut just as much as I can taste ten at a time." Is this true with you? Check out your satiety center now. Has it registered that you have eaten nuts and found them pleasurable?

Cheese. Have you ever at one sitting eaten about four ounces of cheese . . . or five . . . and thought, "I've got to keep cheese out of the house"? Or at a party, thought,

"Let me get away from the cheese table because once I start I have no control"? If you are a cheesaholic, you'll like this tasting experience. Cut a piece of cheese into four one-eighth-ounce slices. Pick up the first piece and wolf it down, chewing very fast and swallowing all at once. Does that seem natural?

Now pick up the next piece and smell it. What kind of cheese is it, a mild, slightly nutty Jarlsberg or a good sharp cheese? Is it a soft, creamy Brie or a hard, crumbly cheddar?

Put the cheese in your mouth and let it . . . that's right . . . s-l-o-w-l-y m-e-l-t. If the cheese is at room temperature this will happen easily and reward you and your 10,000 taste buds with a delicious, full bouquet of flavors and textures.

After this piece has melted, go on to the next one and then the next, making sure to take plenty of time. Try for three minutes per piece. Most people say, "I never really knew what that particular cheese tasted like," and are surprised to find that they intensely like or *dis*like that particular type of cheese!

In these exercises we are showing you that your satiety—or taste center—can register with a very small amount of food. By eating slowly and allowing yourself to get the complete aroma, taste and texture from each bite you will be able to safely sample the "sitting out food" at home or a party without becoming too full to enjoy the more important main dishes. And by now you should be fully aware that since you haven't eaten abnormal quantities of food, you won't gain weight; *can't* gain weight!

One reason that my diet is so successful is that I get

your taste buds working at peak level. This week savor
every bite of food, play with it with your tongue, let
each morsel melt in your mouth before you swallow it.
Make every fork or spoonful of food into the sensuous
experience it is meant to be.

STEP THREE

Eat One Food at a Time in Order of Preference

You may not have noticed this, but most Overeaters
save the best for last. Fat people wade through masses
of foods they are actually indifferent to to get to the reward—the food they really want.

True Thins don't do that. They eat the foods they find
most desirable first and so don't load their bodies with
a lot of *duty* calories. Duty calories will make you fat
because they force you to overeat to get to the foods
that are necessary to your dining pleasure. When you
sit down to dinner tonight, look at your plate and ask
yourself, "Which food would I fight for?" Eat that first,
and do not return to it. After you have eaten all you
want of your first choice, proceed to your second (remembering that you can't go back to any food), and then your
other choices, in order of preference. For example, if
you have a steak, baked potato, salad and rolls on your
plate, which one would you want first? Steak? Potato?
Rolls? Salad? You probably wouldn't choose the salad as
your *first,* "favorite" choice, but isn't that what you *usually* start with? And maybe it isn't the steak either. You
could have eaten the steak first in the past because it
was the most expensive item on the plate and you think
you have to get your money's worth out of the meal.

Perhaps what you would really like is the hot rolls with butter or the baked potato. If so, eat and enjoy them to their fullest before proceeding to the other items on your plate.

You're going to have a number of surprises in store for you this week as you find out what you want the most. I think this is one of the most delightful aspects of my diet, this opportunity to stimulate yourself to analyze your true food preferences and then give yourself permission to eat your favorite foods to your heart's content, instead of plodding through those boring duty foods.

STEP FOUR

Eat Slowly

All diets tell you to eat slowly, but I'm going to ask you to do more than that. This week you are to eat slowly for ten minutes, putting your fork down between each bite, and then after the ten minutes are up, *stop for five minutes.*

Read the newspaper if you like. Talk to your spouse and the children. Leave the table if you wish. Make a phone call. Do anything you please *except* eat.

After five minutes have elapsed you may resume eating (making sure to put your fork down between each bite), and continue until you are full.

The *minimum* amount of time you are allowed to take per meal is twenty minutes. For faster weight loss, you should try to stretch your dining time to forty minutes or more.

Why is it so important to take a break after eating for ten minutes? Because it takes twenty minutes or more for your hypothalamus to register fullness and satiety.

The hypothalamus (Figure 1) is a part of the brain located near the back of the lower part of your skull. This area has many receptor centers, one of which registers *fullness* and the other *taste satisfaction* (satiety).

Figure 1
HYPOTHALAMUS
Takes 20 Minutes to Register

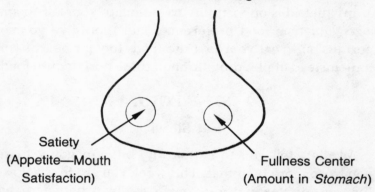

Satiety
(Appetite—Mouth
Satisfaction)

Fullness Center
(Amount in *Stomach*)

Both of these centers must register for you to have a satisfying eating experience. Therefore, you must eat slowly to allow time for the signals that are released when you start to eat to travel up to the brain and signal to the fullness center in your hypothalamus that you have eaten enough to be comfortably full. If you gulp your food, you are going to eat an extra large quantity before your fullness center gets the chance to tell you you have had enough; you will have gobbled down extra food you didn't want or need to feel happily full, and that extra food will go straight to—you guessed it—fat.

But feeling full is only half of your goal. Have you ever eaten a large quantity of food such as a bunch of raw celery or a large diet salad without dressing and felt full . . . but dissatisfied? That is because your fullness center had registered all right, but your satiety center had not.

I'm sure you have found yourself saying when you have dieted before, "I'm full but I still want something to eat!" Well, of *course* you do!

Now think of the times when you have eaten a small quantity of something you really wanted . . . how contented you felt . . . comfortable and satisfied. That's because your satiety center registered.

Both centers in the hypothalamus must register or you are going to be driven to eat destructively and gain weight.

STEP FIVE

Drink Six 10-ounce Glasses of Water a Day

I suggest you drink two glasses of water in the morning, three in the afternoon and one in the evening. The reason for this spacing is to keep the body cells hydrated. You see, you usually lose two pounds of water weight overnight through respiration, perspiration and urination. When you wake up, your body is dehydrated, and it is necessary to replace that water for your cells to be able to function efficiently. What does all this have to do with weight loss?

Unless your cells are kept hydrated, they can't burn off fat properly. If you don't drink at least 60 ounces of water a day, you will lose only half as much weight per week.

No other liquid is an acceptable substitute for the water. Iced tea doesn't count. Diet sodas don't count. Coffee doesn't count. Only water will have the miraculous effect of hydrating your body cells completely and sparking high-powered Fat-Burn-Out.

I personally prefer sipping ice water throughout the day, but many people who have taken my course think room temperature water is more pleasant. You will have to experiment with both and make up your own mind about which you like better. This will also be true about the *type* of water you will be drinking. Some people get hooked on various commercial bottled waters. I don't care what kind of water you drink as long as you drink a minimum of 60 ounces a day.

I realize that some of you have become so used to getting your necessary daily liquids from artificial, "civilized" sources, that you don't even remember what water tastes like, but if you want to lose those hated extra pounds, you are going to have to do what your primitive ancestors did—drink lots of water. Eventually you will enjoy drinking water and your thinning body will crave it.

You may also drink coffee, tea and diet sodas, of course, but you must *never* consider these beverages acceptable substitutes for water, for they aren't!

I do want to sound one note of caution. Don't try to drink all or most of your day's quota of water in one sitting to "get it over with." Not only would doing so probably make you feel sick, but such a practice would be self-defeating. You need to keep your cells fully hydrated *throughout* the day, not just for a few hours, to attain maximum weight loss.

STEP SIX

Fill Out Every Section of Your Food Sheets Daily

Added to the end of this chapter are seven blank Food Sheets. (Again, as mentioned earlier in this book, if you want to keep these charts confidential, put them through a duplicating machine and then store the sheets in a private file.) These must be filled in, in detail, every time you eat something. For example, let's say you reached HUNGER LEVEL 3 at 12:30 P.M. and ate a cheeseburger and french fries, all of which took you (including that all-important five-minute break) twenty minutes to consume. You would enter this information on your Food Sheet thusly:

TIME OF DAY	LEVEL OF HUNGER	FOOD EATEN AND AMOUNT	TIME TAKEN TO EAT
12:30 p.m.	#3	1 cheeseburger 1 order of french fries	20 min.

At the bottom of the page, where you see the words 5 MIN. BREAK, you would make a check mark indicating you had taken the required five-minute rest after the first ten minutes of eating:

5 MIN. BREAK √

If you drank one of your 10-ounce glasses of water at lunch, make that notation with a check mark after the word WATER at the bottom of the Food Sheet:

WATER √

Your dinner that day will be entered in exactly the same way:

TIME OF DAY	LEVEL OF HUNGER	FOOD EATEN AND AMOUNT	TIME TAKEN TO EAT
8:00 p.m.	*#3*	*½ sliced tomato* *New York strip steak* *1 browned potato* *¼ cup cooked carrots* *1 roll with butter*	*40 min.*

Figure 2 shows what your completed Food Sheet for the day, including your 60 ounces of water, would look like.

TIME OF DAY	LEVEL OF HUNGER	FOOD EATEN AND AMOUNT	TIME TAKEN TO EAT
12:30 p.m.	#3	1 cheeseburger 1 order of french fries	20 min.
8:00 p.m.	#3	½ sliced tomato New York strip steak 1 browned potato ¼ cup cooked carrots 1 roll with butter	40 min.

5 MIN. BREAK √ √

WATER √ √ √ √ √ √

Figure 2

There are several reasons why filling out your Food Sheets will help you lose weight:

1. Having to enter your hunger level will make you analyze whether you are actually at HUNGER LEVEL 3 or still at HUNGER LEVEL 2, and keep you from eating at those times when your body can't burn off fat.

2. Teach you your individual hunger pattern—the number of times a day and when they occur that are normal for you to experience true hunger (three-time-a-day hunger, two-time-a-day hunger, one-time-a-day hunger).

3. Show you WHY if you don't lose weight during that week. For example, take a look at one of Mary Ann's Food Sheets (Figure 3). When Mary Ann enrolled in my Naturally Slim course she was a large woman with about 70 pounds to lose. When she returned after the first week she had lost only 1 pound, while everyone else in her class had lost 4 to 9 pounds! Naturally she was very disappointed and thought my diet was "no good." Mary Ann said, "Sandra, I don't want to hurt your feelings, but I knew that I couldn't lose weight eating Mexican food and salad dressing." She had eaten a piece of diet bread with margarine even though she wasn't hungry!

"Mary Ann," I said, "why did you eat that toast every day when you *knew* you were at HUNGER LEVEL 1?"

"Well, my husband is worried that if I don't eat a little something in the morning I'll get weak, so I didn't want to upset him," she admitted sheepishly. "I thought since it was low calorie, it wouldn't cause any problem."

"Mary Ann, you obviously don't have morning hunger—your Food Sheets show that clearly—so please don't eat that diet toast and margarine next week, and I promise you, you'll lose weight."

TIME OF DAY	LEVEL OF HUNGER	FOOD EATEN AND AMOUNT	TIME TAKEN TO EAT
7:30 a.m.	1	1 piece of diet toast and 1 teaspoon of diet margarine	20 min.
1:00 p.m.	3	grilled cheese sandwich 6 french fries	38 min.
7:15 p.m.	3	1 beef taco 1 cheese enchilada salad (small)	45 min.

5 MIN. BREAK √ √ √
WATER √ √ √ √ √ √

Figure 3

Mary Ann was amazed to find when she returned the following week that she had lost 7 pounds, a total of 8 pounds for two weeks. From then on she ate only at HUNGER LEVEL 3 and lost her extra 70 pounds while eating Mexican foods and rich salad dressings every time she was hungry for them.

Memories are unreliable. Food Sheets aren't. Can you tell from the Food Sheet in Figure 4 why this person did not lose weight that day?

If you said she shouldn't have had a frozen daiquiri, you were right, *not* because it was an alcoholic beverage, but because that beverage contained sugar. If she had had a whiskey and soda or martini, she would have lost weight that day in spite of eating rolls, chowder and lobster!

See if you can analyze the Food Sheet in Figure 5.

If you guessed that the mistake this dieter made that cost him no weight loss that day was in eating the cheese and crackers at HUNGER LEVEL 2, you were right. The big Chinese dinner eaten at HUNGER LEVEL 3 didn't put an ounce on him because his body was ready at 6:00 to assimilate anything he ate!

STEP SEVEN

Be Patient with Yourself

While the Dallas Doctors' Diet isn't a deprivation diet, it is a very *different* one from any you have ever known. Initially your body will be baffled that you aren't eating three meals a day at familiar times. Also, you will feel psychologically confused and uncomfortable at having familiar rituals taken away from you. Experts say that it takes twenty-one days for human beings to become com-

TIME OF DAY	LEVEL OF HUNGER	FOOD EATEN AND AMOUNT	TIME TAKEN TO EAT
11:30	*#3*	*1 turkey pot pie* *1 roll with butter* *½ apple*	*30 min.*
7:30	*#3*	*1 frozen daiquiri* *1 cup of New England clam chowder* *1 small broiled lobster with butter* *fresh asparagus*	*30 min.*

5 MIN. BREAK   X X

WATER X X X X X X

Figure 4

TIME OF DAY	LEVEL OF HUNGER	FOOD EATEN AND AMOUNT	TIME TAKEN TO EAT
10:30 a.m.	*#2*	*2 crackers and cheese*	*5 min.*
6:00 p.m.	*#3*	*1 egg roll egg drop soup chicken chow mein with rice and noodles 1 fortune cookie*	*30 min.*

5 MIN. BREAK   X X
WATER   XXXXXX

Figure 5

fortable with a new eating pattern, so be patient with yourself. Don't panic if your head sends out signals that it is "time to eat because it is twelve noon," while your body is also telling you "I'm not hungry yet." It won't be long before eating only when you are hungry will be the normal, familiar way for your body and mind to deal with food.

Also, please be patient with yourself if you make mistakes in the beginning, such as thinking you are at HUNGER LEVEL 3 when you are still at HUNGER LEVEL 2. Many people are slow to discern the differences in hunger levels. Time and experience will remedy these errors in judgment. It took Dr. Agnew nearly three weeks to clearly judge his personal hunger pattern, *but* he still lost weight during that three weeks and, once he was able to tell a hundred percent of the time when he had reached LEVEL 3, he almost doubled his weekly weight loss.

Now a couple of last reminders as you prepare to start your first week on the Dallas Doctors' Diet. As is not the case with other diets, the weight you lose this week will not be water weight, but *fat*. If you think about it, how *could* you be losing water when you're drinking so much?

And unlike other diets that promise you huge instantaneous weight losses ("You will lose 20 pounds and inches in three days"), the Dallas Doctors' Diet offers you no imaginary miracles; but you will lose a healthy amount of weight each week and, most importantly, that weight *will never return* as long as you continue to eat only when hungry and drink your water.

DR. WAYNE AGNEW'S CAPSULE COMMENTS:
The most controversial aspect of this diet is that it dis-

putes the deeply entrenched belief of the medical and nutritional communities that breakfast is the most important
meal of the day. We all have heard the admonition "eat
breakfast like a king, lunch like a queen and dinner like a
pauper." For some people (approximately 5%) this is sound
advice, but for 95% of the population, eating 300 to 1,500
calories of food that the body is unable to utilize efficiently
on the off chance that you MIGHT get hungry later or
MIGHT need some food energy later just doesn't make
sense. The first few days I went without breakfast, however,
I will admit to you I was a little concerned. What if I became
tired during surgery? What if I became too "weak" to keep
up my hectic morning pace of rounds, consultations and
appointments? What if my brain didn't stay sharp enough
to make correct diagnoses and decisions? In many jobs
there is a sizable margin for error, but a physician doesn't
have that luxury.

My concerns were shortlived. My energy level, brain function and efficiency actually increased once my body was
freed of the burden of trying to absorb a breakfast it wasn't
ready or able to turn into body fuel. You are likely to have
the same pleasant surprise that I did—feeling better without
breakfast than with it.

So saying, I should warn you that if you are one of the
rare individuals who experience dizziness, severe headache
or sudden, unexplained feelings of intense anxiety or depression that you think could be caused by not having had
breakfast, then eat one-half to one ounce of cheese or a
tablespoon of peanut butter slowly. If your symptoms disappear shortly thereafter, you MAY have had a low blood-
sugar reaction, and I would suggest that you see your physician before proceeding further on this diet. I might point
out, however, that although several thousand people have

followed Sandra Breithaupt's instructions and not eaten breakfast for three days in a row, NO ONE has ever reported symptoms of a low blood-sugar-level reaction. Ruth Thomas, the Naturally Slim instructor in Arlington, Texas, and I worked with individuals who had been diagnosed as having hypoglycemia, and they didn't have any trouble that would suggest low blood-sugar levels throughout the day.

The interactions of the human body are myriad. One of the most important points that Sandra makes is the importance of eating slowly so that there is time for the hypothalamus to tell you you are full. Her other point about the hypothalamus—that both the fullness and satiety centers must register—is equally valid and should be kept in mind when planning each meal.

To recapitulate, this week on the Dallas Doctors' Diet, you are to:

- go without breakfast the first three mornings . . .
- eat only when at HUNGER LEVEL 3 . . .
- eat anything you want (with the exceptions of fruit and vegetable juices, cereals, milk and sweets), but *taste* your food . . .
- eat in order of preference; do not return to any food . . .
- eat slowly for ten minutes, putting your fork down between each bite, and then stop for five minutes . . .
- spend a minimum of twenty minutes at each meal; try for forty . . .
- drink six 10-ounce glasses of water per day . . .
- fill in your Food Sheet immediately after each meal . . .
- be patient with yourself. There is an inevitable period of confusion—of trial and error—and a degree of discomfort at having familiar habits altered is to be expected.

TIME OF DAY	LEVEL OF HUNGER	FOOD EATEN AND AMOUNT	TIME TAKEN TO EAT
		5 MIN. BREAK _____ WATER _____	

TIME OF DAY	LEVEL OF HUNGER	FOOD EATEN AND AMOUNT	TIME TAKEN TO EAT
		5 MIN. BREAK _____ WATER _____	

TIME OF DAY	LEVEL OF HUNGER	FOOD EATEN AND AMOUNT	TIME TAKEN TO EAT
		5 MIN. BREAK _____ WATER _____	

TIME OF DAY	LEVEL OF HUNGER	FOOD EATEN AND AMOUNT	TIME TAKEN TO EAT
		5 MIN. BREAK _____	
		WATER _____	

TIME OF DAY	LEVEL OF HUNGER	FOOD EATEN AND AMOUNT	TIME TAKEN TO EAT
		5 MIN. BREAK _____	
		WATER _____	

TIME OF DAY	LEVEL OF HUNGER	FOOD EATEN AND AMOUNT	TIME TAKEN TO EAT
		5 MIN. BREAK _____ WATER _____	

TIME OF DAY	LEVEL OF HUNTER	FOOD EATEN AND AMOUNT	TIME TAKEN TO EAT
		5 MIN. BREAK _____ WATER _____	

5

THE
DALLAS DOCTORS'
WEEK ONE

THE DALLAS DOCTORS were weighing in to see the results of their first week on my diet:

Dr. Cliff Daniel, who started the program at 200 pounds, tonight weighs 196 pounds. Good.

Dr. Mike Mendelson's weight last week was 224 pounds; one week later it is 213 pounds. Superb! An 11-pound weight loss.

Dr. Bill Pirtle has gone from 217 to 210½ pounds, a 6½-pound loss. Excellent.

Dr. Jack Wilson, who'd weighed in at 237½ pounds last week is now at 230 pounds. Wonderful.

Dr. Sandy Reitman, who had started the program at 198, weighed in at 192¾ pounds. Very good.

Dr. Jerry Bane has gone from 191 pounds down to 186. Another good result.

I looked around at my "pupils." "You all did really well this week, which I know must have been difficult for you. It is very hard to change habits of many years' standing, but each of you has taken a giant step in the direction of life-long thinness. A couple of you didn't lose as much weight as I thought you could have, so we will have to try to find out where you went wrong. Did any of you have trouble going without breakfast for the first three days? Cliff?"

"I thought it would be a real problem to get up and not have cereal or something before going to work. We all grew up believing something bad would happen if we didn't eat a big breakfast, we'd fail our exams or whatever. But to my surprise, I found out that eating a very hearty breakfast had been making me sleepy, and worst of all, it had been making me hungry again right away. I did just fine without breakfast."

"Mike, you never eat breakfast, so I'll pass you by on this one. Bill?"

"I didn't find it difficult, but then I didn't expect to."

"Jack?"

"It wasn't easy when I saw the jelly doughnuts my kids were eating, but I got through it."

"Sandy?"

"Like Cliff, I always thought that *you have to eat breakfast.* I thought if you were upset or nervous in the morning it was because you hadn't eaten a good breakfast. I expected to be the grouchiest, most difficult person on earth, but I stayed even-tempered and wasn't hungry. I don't think I'm a breakfast person."

"Jerry, did you find it difficult to go without breakfast for three mornings?"

"No, because I didn't. I *have* to eat breakfast. I wouldn't dare operate otherwise. If you're going to do strenuous work like surgery, you gotta eat a big breakfast. I especially need my milk. I could never risk not being able to do my best in surgery."

"Milk!" Mike Mendelson looked astonished. "What are you doing drinking milk at your age, Jerry?"

"Why shouldn't I drink milk? What's wrong with it?"

"I've read that after six years of age many people gradually stop producing the enzyme that is necessary to digest milk," I said. "Is that so, Mike?"

"That's right. That's exactly right."

Wayne spoke up. "I understand your breakfast fears, Jerry, but I guess you are aware that I also have a heavy morning surgery schedule, and I've learned that I have *more* stamina and my mind is sharper if I don't eat breakfast. I wish you would try, just a couple of times in a row, to go without eating in the morning to see if that's true for you too. After all, one of the nurses can always get you something if you feel your energy dipping."

"That's true. All right. I might try it on Saturday and Sunday when I'm not on call."

"I would appreciate that, Jerry," I said. "You may turn out to be in the five-percent group of people who should eat breakfast because that's normal for their body chemistry, but if you aren't, eating breakfast will impede your weight loss.

"Now, what did all of you find out about your food tastes when you started eating in order of preference?"

"I was surprised to discover that I liked beef better than I thought I did," Cliff Daniel said. "I've always been a carbohydrate sort of person, and we haven't eaten much meat since the first consumer boycott of the cattle raisers way back made the prices shoot up, but when I looked at my dinner plate several times this week and saw that beef, I said 'I really *want* some of this stuff!' "

"I now know that my favorite food is potatoes," Bill Pirtle said. "That's all I ate one night . . . just fried potatoes. And another night my first choice was a big bowl of blackeyed peas, which I just kept eating until I was full. Before I would have eaten all the rest of the dinner to get the right to eat the french fries or blackeyed peas or whatever I wanted the most."

"Every one of you marked on your EATING PROFILE forms that you were fast eaters. Were you able to slow down this week?"

Mike Mendelson laughed. "I drove people crazy. I don't think Brody will go out to eat with me again. We had all gone sailing and then stopped off in this place to eat. They were all making fun of me, you know, but I had already started to lose a lot of weight, so I said, 'Well, let me show you how to eat. You take a little . . . you look at the food . . . you smell it . . . you put a little in your mouth and chew it slowly . . . then you take another little piece. . . .' I drove them crazy. It took me God knows how long just to eat one burrito. Brody's wife said, 'Mendelson, don't you think it's time to get out of here?' I said, 'You wanted to know how I'm eating, right? It's just the way you're supposed to eat.' We ate for about three hours there."

Sandy Reitman chimed in, "I liked putting my fork down between bites. It was very effective. After each bite I'd put it down and take time to enjoy the food. I hadn't noticed before that a lot of overweight people tend to be working on the next twelve bites while they're eating that first bite."

Jack Wilson commented, "My wife just loves this program because I've started to sit around now and talk to her at meals; before when I was through eating, I got up. I was antsy; ready to go."

I went on to the next step. "Did anyone have trouble drinking the water?"

Jack Wilson grimaced. "I had to choke it down, but I drank it all."

"Jerry?"

"This was the easiest part of the diet this week for me. I run a lot, and in Texas if you run you get dehydrated. So I drink water all the time. I don't drink Cokes and root beers and that sort of thing, just tap water; and I'm sure I drink more than sixty ounces a day. Normally I drink eight or ten glasses a day, and in the summertime even more."

Cliff reported, "I never drank water before this diet . . . not *pure* water. Only in coffee or tea. This is quite a change. I'm finding this very difficult."

Sandy Reitman seemed a bit sheepish. "Look, I haven't had sixty ounces of water in forty years of my life. It's horrible. I'm a tea drinker. I can't drink all this water. Two or three glasses a day is the best I've been able to do."

"I hope you will keep trying, Sandy, because the water is so important. If you don't drink at least six ten-ounce glasses a day, you will lose only HALF as much weight.

"Did all of you fill in your Food Sheets?"

Everyone nodded "yes."

"Did you find it was difficult to tell when you had reached HUNGER LEVEL 3?"

Everyone again nodded "yes."

"That isn't surprising, for learning to identify the differences between appetite and hunger takes time."

Cliff said, "I'm still having some difficulty in this area. I have made one discovery: apparently I have always eaten to *keep* from being hungry. When I finally let myself become hungry, around the end of the week, I finally understood what you mean by HUNGER LEVEL 3."

"I found myself eating when I wasn't fully hungry yet," concurred Bill Pirtle, "because I was afraid I would be hungry two hours later. I think much of the week I ate before I was quite at HUNGER LEVEL 3."

"Your Food Sheets reflect your observations. Cliff, I think you will find next week that you can lose a little faster if you wait until you are *sure* you are at HUNGER LEVEL 3 before eating. You might even allow yourself to get to HUNGER LEVEL 4 just once so that you get a full understanding of what overhunger feels like. This can help you evaluate whether or not you have reached real hunger [(LEVEL 3)] in the future. Your Food Sheets indicate, Cliff and Bill, that you have two-time-a-day hunger patterns, so that information should also help you make some educated guesses about the times of day you are most likely to reach full hunger.

"Mike, you very clearly have one-time-a-day hunger, but the fact that your schedule has you eating that meal so late at night may cause you some snacking and binging problems. The Save Your Hunger Technique that is part of Week Two's instruction plan should help you deal with this.

"Jack, I suspect that you may find that you have two-time-a-day hunger some days and others only one-time-a-day hunger. But it will be another week or so before the patterns that are normal for you will emerge clearly.

"Sandy, you seem to have two-time-a-day hunger, and with the exception of not drinking enough water, you did splendidly this week adjusting yourself to this diet. And I'm sure you noticed that your drinking a martini every night before dinner didn't slow down your Fat-Burn-Out mechanism."

"Frankly, that surprised me. I wasn't *about* to miss my nightly martini, but I was sure I would pay for it on the scales. When I hit the house, the first thing I do is sit down with the mail and newspaper and have a martini. Everybody in my family except the dogs can make my martini. It's a nice skill to have. Takes a second. And that's my sort of period to unwind from the hospital mentality to Daddy, home, husband mentality and it's just gotten built into the five, five-thirty, six o'clock spot."

"Just be sure, Sandy, that you're always at HUNGER LEVEL 3 when you drink your martini, and it won't cost you any weight loss.

"Jerry, you were the best water drinker of the group, but until you try going without breakfast to see if you have three-time-a-day hunger or one of the more common eating patterns, you won't be able to achieve your full potential on this diet. But in spite of the fact that you ate breakfast and sneaked in a dessert this week, you still managed to lose five pounds, which shows that you are an excellent candidate for this program.

"All in all, I think every one of you has made a splendid start on your desire to lose your excess weight and keep it off forever. Do you *like* the diet?"

"You bet," Dr. Jack Wilson said. "This is the easiest way I've ever found to lose weight. It's so easy it's amazing."

Dr. Sandy Reitman agreed. "I was totally able to disregard calorie content, the quality of foods. That has always been too much busy work for me. I've stopped carrying calorie books in my pocket. I've stopped weighing foods. This week I disregarded cholesterol, I disregarded fats, I disregarded balanced meals. I ignored all that stuff and ate foods that turned me on and lost five and a half pounds! This is wonderful."

"Bill?"

"This being able to eat basically what I want and still lose weight has really impressed me," Dr. Bill Pirtle said.

"I have a continuous spectrum of clothes . . . small, medium and large; I throw them out periodically and then always have to go buy them back. This is the first diet I've ever been on that has made me think it will be possible to have just one size clothes in my closet," commented Dr. Cliff Daniel.

Dr. Jerry Bane offered, "This is so much easier than eating all that rabbit food that is the base of most diet programs. I *enjoy* fresh fruits and vegetables and I eat a lot of them, but I can't stand the thought of having to eat *just* that and nothing else. This is something I may be able to get comfortable with and stay with."

Dr. Mike Mendelson was enthusiastic. "When I eat, I really eat. I eat it all, I eat it *all.* I eat anything and everything. I will admit to you, I was skeptical that I could eat a large variety of foods and lose weight at the same time, but I took off eleven pounds in this first week by eating in this new way. I'm impressed."

DR. WAYNE AGNEW'S CAPSULE COMMENTS:

The Dallas Doctors' respective weight losses this week were:

     Dr. Jerry Bane—5 pounds
     Dr. Cliff Daniel—4 pounds
     Dr. Mike Mendelson—11 pounds

Dr. Bill Pirtle—6½ pounds

Dr. Sandy Reitman—5¼ pounds

Dr. Jack Wilson—7½ pounds

These figures are excellent, but duplicable on other diet regimens. What makes the Dallas Doctors' results so unique is that they reduced their weight while continuing to eat non-diet foods, and they learned a great deal about how their bodies were meant to function in respect to hunger patterns (i.e., one-time-a-day hunger, two-time-a-day hunger, three-time-a-day hunger, two-time-a-day hunger some days/one-time-a-day hunger others), food preferences, eating habits and the amounts and types of food that are necessary to make them feel both full and emotionally satisfied.

Most people go a lifetime without gaining this knowledge about themselves.

One thing I'm sure you, the reader, noticed, was that the Dallas Doctors made mistakes this week in judging when they had reached HUNGER LEVEL 3. They resisted (except for Dr. Jerry Bane) drinking their six 10-ounce glasses of water a day, and they had to consciously work on eating more slowly and making decisions about what to eat. You will probably have these same difficulties in your first week on the 3D, as we have nicknamed this program. But be patient. As you follow the Dallas Doctors through this program you will see that every week it gets easier and easier. This is because, as Sandra Breithaupt so astutely pointed out, it takes approximately twenty-one days for any new form of behavior, even a highly pleasurable one, to become a comfortable habit. Also, the 3D requires more *mental* attention than any other diet I have worked with. Usually we doctors hand out printed sheets of "do" and "don't" foods to patients along with instructions on quantities (meager!) and meal-scheduling that are so inflexible that the patient isn't involved in any thinking processes while he or she is dieting. Patients quickly become miserable in these diet strait jackets, of course, which explains why they seldom stay in them for any length of time.

The Dallas Doctors' Diet removes the diet strait jackets that you have struggled against so strongly in the past, but, because it is a thinking person's diet, it will require input from you: concentration; a degree of intelligence; willingness to shed your old, fat-accumulating ways of eating, and the patience to go through the minor trials and errors that are inescapable during the early weeks of the 3D program.

After a lifetime of fighting obesity, I was willing, even *eager* to go through the adjustments that the Dallas Doctors' Diet requires so that I could become a True Thin and savor the pleasures of eating my favorite foods without guilt or fear.

I also found the process of discovering what my body's normal hunger patterns actually are an intellectually interesting one. My six Dallas colleagues, as you can see from the first week's report, are also finding the program a stimulating one, and well worth taking their very valuable time and energies to continue to explore. I hope you will do the same.

6

WEEK TWO
OF THE
DALLAS DOCTORS'
DIET

WHEN I HAVE interviewed Overeaters, I have often found that they are burdened with an impressive number of *beliefs* about food—beliefs they have never thought to question. But True Thins, although they had been told various truisms about food when they were growing up, either ignored them or tested them out and discarded them because they weren't applicable to their personal hunger patterns.

Most Overeaters believe the following statements are true; True Thins know they are false. Do you accept these myths?

• I should eat a hearty breakfast. It will start the day off right.

- I should eat three meals a day.
- I should eat well-balanced meals.
- I should clean my plate.
- I should save the best for last.
- Sweets give you quick energy.
- I shouldn't skip meals.
- I'll get sick if I don't eat "regularly."

Dr. Bill Pirtle spoke up. "I think we all have learned enough in the last week to realize that these statements are generally untrue and destructive to our attempts to keep our weight down. But Sandra, I am a bit disturbed by the implication that eating well-balanced meals isn't important. It is. We need the nutrients from fruits, vegetables and protein foods to have healthy bodies."

"True, Bill, but there's no validity to the theory that you have to get *all* your nutrients at *every* meal. What's wrong with eating only fish and fresh fruit at one meal and only potatoes and bread at another? The nutrient tally at the end of that day will still be a good one."

"Yes, *if* people choose from those food groups. But aren't they just as likely, when you tell them to eat anything they want, to pick pizza and Twinkies?"

"Initially yes, but as people learn to identify the messages their bodies are giving them, they will eat enough nutritious foods during the span of a week, say, to stay healthy. This is because your body's desire for healthier, less rich foods will transmit the appropriate signals to your appetite control center. I was just going over the Food Sheets of a woman in one of my Shreveport classes who is a good example of how your body will regulate itself when given the chance. Terry ate mostly rich foods for three days, things like fettuccini Alfredo, croissants, Welsh rarebit and duck à l'orange, and then suddenly on the Food Sheets I could see that she had switched her tastes completely. At one meal she had about five fruits and a bran muffin and at another meal she ate only fresh green beans, a tomato and some boiled shrimp."

"I haven't been eating *any* balanced meals or nutritious ones," Jack Wilson objected.

"Oh, but you have, Jack. Take a look at your Food Sheet for Thursday. For lunch you had vegetable soup, cheese and crackers. At dinner you ate ham, squash and an apple. Why did you choose those particular foods?"

"Because my wife had cooked them, I guess."

"But if they hadn't tasted good to you, would you have settled for those selections?"

"Hell no. I'd have said, 'Bring on some good stuff,' or gone out for a hamburger."

"Exactly."

Dr. Jerry Bane observed, "They've shown in numerous studies that when you let babies and small children eat anything they want, they may eat all ice cream one day, but the next they will go for vegetables or fruits or whatever and will end up having eaten mostly 'good' foods over a period of several days. I agree that it is nice but not necessary to always eat completely balanced meals."

"Does everyone accept that I SHOULD EAT A HEARTY BREAKFAST, I SHOULD EAT THREE MEALS A DAY, I SHOULD EAT WELL-BALANCED MEALS, I SHOULD CLEAN MY PLATE, I SHOULD SAVE THE BEST FOR LAST, SWEETS GIVE YOU QUICK ENERGY, I SHOULDN'T SKIP MEALS and I'LL GET SICK IF I DON'T EAT 'REGULARLY' are all food myths? Good. The reason I'm making such a point of the fact that you have been cherishing a number of incorrect beliefs about eating, is that *mindlessly acting on these beliefs has contributed to your becoming fat.*

"Doctor Agnew has pointed out that this is a thinking

person's diet and if you are going to be successful at losing weight you will have to ask yourself every time you are about to eat something, 'Why am I eating this now?' The only valid answer is 'because I am hungry and this is the food I am hungry for.' Can you name any other false food beliefs?"

"You shouldn't eat before going to bed," Mike Mendelson contributed. "I do a lot of my work at night, so when I hit home it's eleven o'clock, eleven-thirty. Carole's always got a paper and she's reading it and I come in and see that she's got something warming on the stove and I just go and take whatever's there, eat it and just go right to sleep, and I haven't suffered any ill effects from this. I don't have any trouble getting to sleep and don't have any digestive problems, and since I'm a gastroenterologist I would be sure to pick up on that."

"Any other food myths?"

"You have to eat a hot meal every day," said Cliff Daniel. "I happen to *like* a hot main course at dinner, but there is no valid health reason to insist that each meal or any meal include hot foods."

"Another belief we tell ourselves is that if you pay for it, you have to eat it," suggested Sandy Reitman.

"And if it's *free* you have to eat it," said Mike Mendelson. "I have a lotta trouble turning down free food. Free *anything*, I'm ready to jump on it. I'm very frugal. I would *never* spend money for myself for lunch, for instance. *Never*. But I go to Arlington Community Hospital and eat lunch there because it's free. It's a *nice* meal, a *very* nice meal, but that's not why I eat it. I eat it because it's free. It was hard passing that free lunch up last week. At least you've made me realize I was eating lunch for a reason other than being hungry."

"Another false belief is that if someone goes to all that trouble to fix it, you have to eat it," Dr. Agnew threw in. "I used to eat a lot of dishes I didn't like too much or wasn't hungry for just because I was afraid I'd hurt Wanda's feelings if I didn't. But I don't do that anymore and Wanda's feelings aren't bruised if I don't like something as much as she does. I'm not a bad person if I'm not turned on by cauliflower, and she's not a better person than I am if she loves cauliflower."

"But it does help to have the cook's understanding, Wayne," Cliff Daniel pointed out. "Myrtle has helped a lot by recognizing the principles of this diet. If she had been rigid and said 'you've got to eat what I've prepared,' this last week would have been difficult. To be honest, when I first got started, there *was* a little bit of a problem because I didn't know what I was hungry for until I was at that point, and it was rarely what she had fixed. How was she supposed to have guessed? Fortunately I didn't get angry with her for not anticipating my needs, and she didn't get angry with me for not always eating everything she had cooked. She was really very flexible. The spouse has to be pretty sympathetic. She has to understand that there's a good reason for that pattern of eating, that if you don't eat what you're hungry for you don't get satisfied. If she can accept that, it's easier to accept that the person trying to lose weight is not going to eat at the same time they always ate. Or eat the same foods. I suspect that the fact that Myrtle is what you call a True Thin makes her more supportive. She's always eaten only the foods she wants and thinks I have that same right."

"You have been telling yourselves things about food and eating that are not so. This is a major reason why you have developed into Overeaters. So INSTRUCTION

NUMBER ONE this week is: *Become aware of and banish any destructive food myths.*

INSTRUCTION NUMBER TWO is: *Learn to recognize and resist 'flirt' foods.*

Flirt foods are tempting foods that you come across by accident—foods that can lure you into unplanned, unnecessary eating. Passing a hot dog vendor's cart, for example, or catching sight of an ice-cream parlor, smelling the wonderful odors emanating from a bakery exhaust fan, seeing food sitting out, noticing previously unthought-of snack items on the grocery store shelves while shopping, seeing a just-out-of-the-oven pizza in a pizza store window, smelling the popping corn in the lobby of the movie theater.

"You are not actually hungry for flirt foods; what they do is momentarily spark your desire for a pleasurable food experience, and this desire creates a false appetite within you. The key words here are "momentary" and "false," for if you resist the urge to buy and eat the flirt food, if you keep on walking or get away from that food, within minutes you will forget all about it. Since you weren't hungry *before* seeing and smelling the flirt food, you won't be hungry after it's out of range of your eyes and nose.

"If you do eat a flirt food, you will gain weight. This is because flirt foods interfere with your Fat-Burn-Out mechanism. *Any* food, even a low-calorie one, eaten when you're not hungry will put weight on you.

"Flirt foods are not very hard to resist once you understand that (1) you are not actually hungry for them at that moment, and (2) that you can go get them later, when you're at HUNGER LEVEL 3, if you still want them.

"INSTRUCTION NUMBER THREE is: *Become more selective in your food combinations.*

"Overeaters eat what I call Unthinking Combinations, which are two or more foods that you eat together without analyzing if each food is desirable to you. True Thins almost invariably eat Thinking Combinations—two or more foods eaten together because they have been *chosen*. For example, look at this dinner eaten by a True Thin at a cafeteria:

> 2 meat balls
> 1 hush puppy
> the top off the macaroni and cheese
> the inside of a dish of cherry cobbler

"The True Thin didn't wade through the spaghetti to get to the meat balls, the part he really likes, just because meatballs and spaghetti always come together. He also didn't order the fish because he was hungry for the hush puppy that goes with it; he asked for, and got, a single hush puppy. In cafeterias the best part of macaroni and cheese is the top, so our True Thin went, as Jack Wilson says, right for 'the good stuff' and ignored the tasteless, starchy macaroni. The same was true of the cherry cobbler. The cherry part was good, the crust soggy and uninteresting, so the True Thin ignored the fact that 'you can't have a cobbler without a crust' and ate only 'the good stuff.'

"Are you getting the idea?

"Here are a few more examples of Unthinking Combinations that can put weight on the Overeater if he or she is eating one to get the other:

> chips and dip
> cheese and crackers

frankfurter with bun
hot fudge sundae

"Last week I had in a class an Overeater who for years
had been eating chips because she likes the guacomole
dip at her favorite restaurant. Now she just takes a spoon,
scoops up the dip, and leaves the chips in the basket
instead of letting them end up on her hips in the form
of fat. You will be able to test out cheese and crackers
yourself in a minute, but let's look at that frankfurter
and bun. If you *like* the bun, go ahead and eat it, but a
True Thin would *think,* before eating this combination,
if he or she was eating the bun just because it was the
container for the frankfurter or because it tasted good
on its own. The same holds true for hot fudge sundaes.
Many people eat the ice cream to get to the hot fudge.
What they really want is the chocolate and that's what
they should eat and push aside the ice cream; or, better
yet, just order a dish of hot fudge! *There's nothing wrong
with doing that.*

"To give you a personal example of how I handle food
combinations, when I eat chicken chow mein, I make
sure that I sprinkle some crispy noodles on top of the
dish, but since I find rice uninteresting, I don't eat it. I
do the same thing with gumbo and rice—a popular dish
in Louisiana—and shrimp Creole. But when I was an
Overeater, I dutifully waded through the combined
foods, just because they traditionally go together."

Wayne spoke up. "At Thanksgiving, I always used to
eat turkey and dressing with gravy when what I actually
wanted was the dressing and gravy. It's not that I don't
like turkey, but I prefer it cold in sandwiches. So now I
have the turkey part of Thanksgiving dinner the next

day. I never would have thought that was all right to do until Sandra showed me that eating *any* food you're not absolutely crazy about and have an immediate hunger for just doesn't make sense."

"To show you what I mean, I have prepared taster plates for each of you, which include three one-and-a-half-inch squares of pastrami, two one-eighth-ounce pieces of cheddar cheese, four Escort brand crackers, one tablespoon of mayonnaise and one tablespoon of mustard.

"Crackers. Please pick up one of the crackers and smell it. Last week we smelled food before we ate it and I feel it's a good habit to get into. Now, take a bite and let the cracker melt in your mouth. These are very rich crackers, so you should experience a rich, almost buttery taste. Chew this bite and swallow, then proceed to finish the cracker, taking small bites and enjoying it.

"Take the second cracker and eat it in the same slow manner, allowing the cracker to soften in your mouth before swallowing. Is it giving your 10,000 taste buds tingles of pleasure?

"Pastrami. Next, pick up one of the pieces of pastrami and smell it. Does this 'strong' food have a strong smell? Place the pastrami in your mouth, let it warm up there so that you can taste it fully when you begin to chew it. Now chew it, moving it from one side of your mouth to the other. Have you ever fully tasted pastrami before?

"Combination number one. Now we're going to combine the two flavors and toss in a couple more to test your palate's abilities to discover good, bad and indifferent food combinations.

"Take your third cracker, put some mayonnaise on it, add a piece of pastrami, then a sliver of cheese and eat it. Do these four foods taste terrific together? Did you enjoy the pastrami more by itself or would you have liked it with the mayonnaise but not the cheese? Do you miss being able to taste the buttery flavor of the cracker? Are you just using the cracker as a base for 'the good stuff?' Left to yourself, how would you combine these foods in the future?

"*Combination number two.* Take your last cracker, put the remaining mayonnaise on it, add the pastrami and cheese and then spread a generous dollop of mustard on the top. Eat this combination slowly, moving each bite around in your mouth. Do you notice that the mustard covers up the flavors of the cheese and pastrami? Because mustard and other strong seasonings can dominate foods when used too heavily, Overeaters tend to eat too much in a fruitless quest to taste the foods underneath the seasonings. By the time this course is over, you will have become a finicky eater, choosing only combinations in which *all* the individual parts match up to the whole. I, for example, usually skip the cheese unless it is a very good one, and eat only the crackers, because I love the *crunch* of crackers . . .

"Which brings me to INSTRUCTION NUMBER FOUR: *Find out whether you are a crunchy or soft food lover.*

"You probably don't know whether you need mostly crunchy or mostly soft foods to satisfy you. If you go back and look at your first choices on your Food Sheets, you will get a clue. I'm a crunchy food person. I *have* to get a crunchy experience at each meal or I'm not satisfied. Other people don't feel happy unless they've eaten creamy, soft foods.

"Bill, you may turn out to be a soft food person since you crave potatoes and bananas. This may be true of you, too, Jerry, since on your Eating Profile you listed ice cream, bread, rolls, biscuits and corn bread as favorite foods. Cliff, the foods you gravitate toward tend to fall more in the crunchy/chewy category—beef, chips, salads, apples, corn.

"There is no right or wrong category. Both crunchy and soft are just fine. The reason for learning which you are is that if you don't get a crunchy or soft taste experience in each meal, your unhappy satiety center will clamor for appeasal, thus making you continue to eat on *beyond fullness,* stopping only when you finally come upon a food that satisfies your need for that soft or crunchy sensation.

"INSTRUCTION NUMBER FIVE is: *Use a Save Your Hunger when you need to adapt to others' eating schedules.*

"I want you to listen to, and act upon, your own personal hunger cycle, but there's no need to be a slave to it. If you find yourself at HUNGER LEVEL 3 at eleven-thirty in the morning, for example, but can't go to lunch until one, you can use a Save Your Hunger to lower your hunger level.

"A Save Your Hunger is a tiny amount of protein food that you let melt in your mouth for several minutes before swallowing. Sample Save Your Hungers are:

- one teaspoon of creamy-style peanut butter
- six peanuts eaten very slowly
- a half-ounce of cheese

"A Save Your Hunger is *not* a snack; it is a tool to lower your hunger level from a three to a two-and-a-half. It will take the edge off your hunger just enough for you to be comfortable until the time you want to eat arrives, and it will keep you from eating too fast and overeating.

"Let's say you are going to a dinner party tonight at seven and you ordinarily experience true hunger at six. If you use a Save Your Hunger at six, it will hold you over until you get to the dinner party.

"Or, if you are a one-time-a-day, *evening* hunger person most days but occasionally reach HUNGER LEVEL 3 earlier in the day, then a Save Your Hunger will keep you from binging. Mike, you usually eat only at dinnertime, but on those days that you are tempted by that free lunch, try eating a Save Your Hunger first and see if that doesn't satisfy you enough to ward off the temptation to binge on a lunch you don't want.

"Remember, Save Your Hungers are *not* snacks and are *not* to be used to prevent you from getting hungry. They are only handy tools to enable you to postpone a mealtime or last until mealtime."

"Won't using a Save Your Hunger stop your Fat-Burn-Out cycle?" Dr. Jack Wilson wanted to know.

"It will if you misuse a Save Your Hunger by eating it when you are at HUNGER LEVEL 2, but that's not how it's intended to be used. Eat Save Your Hungers only at HUNGER LEVEL 3. They will lower your hunger level to two-and-a-half and guarantee that you will be back up to a LEVEL 3, not a destructive LEVEL 4, when you sit down to eat your meal.

"Let me show you a Food Sheet with a Save Your Hunger on it." (Figure 6.)

"Now take a look at the Food Sheet of a doctor who awakens every morning at six and starts his hospital rounds at seven." (Figure 7.)

"Try to make a Save Your Hunger stretch eight to ten minutes. This can be done. Any questions?"

TIME OF DAY	LEVEL OF HUNGER	FOOD EATEN AND AMOUNT	TIME TAKEN TO EAT
11:30	*3*	*small chef salad with blue-cheese dressing (about 3 T.)*	*32 min.*
5:30	*3*	*½ oz. of cheese (cut in tiny pieces and allowed to melt in the mouth)*	*12 min.*
8:15	*3*	*3 bites of salad ½ sirloin strip steak ½ baked potato with sour cream and about 1 T. butter 1 bite roll*	*40 min.*

5 MIN. BREAK   XX

WATER   XXXXXX

Figure 6

TIME OF DAY	LEVEL OF HUNGER	FOOD EATEN AND AMOUNT	TIME TAKEN TO EAT
10:30	*3*	*1 tsp. (large) of creamy peanut butter slowly licked*	*10 min.*
12:30	*3*	*lunch of grilled cheese and bacon sandwich cole slaw 3 potato chips pickle*	*21 min.*
6:30	*3*	*roast leg of lamb 1 browned potato green beans melon*	*35 min.*

5 MIN. BREAK X X

WATER X X X X X X

Figure 7

"Can you eat more than one Save Your Hunger?" Dr. Bill Pirtle queried.

"Yes, but please wait a minimum of forty-five minutes between Save Your Hungers. I know you go to a number of banquets, Bill, and the food is often served later than promised. If you've reached HUNGER LEVEL 3 at six-thirty say, and you take a Save Your Hunger to hold you until the seven-thirty banquet, but seven-thirty comes and no food is in sight, by all means eat a few peanuts if you are at HUNGER LEVEL 3. This will keep you from over-drinking or wolfing down hors d'oeuvres you don't want. Just always be on guard against turning a Save Your Hunger into a snack or eating it when you are not at a full HUNGER LEVEL 3.

"Any other questions?"

"When are we going to get to eat sweets?" Jerry Bane asked.

"Next week—Week Three—will be a sweet experience for you, I promise you. This week concentrate on:

1. becoming aware of and banishing destructive food myths;

2. learning to recognize and resist flirt foods;

3. becoming more selective in your food combinations;

4. finding out whether you are a crunchy or soft food lover;

5. using Save Your Hungers when you need to adapt to others' eating schedules."

DR. WAYNE AGNEW'S CAPSULE COMMENTS:

Save Your Hungers, judiciously used, can make all the difference in how you adjust to the Dallas Doctors' Diet.

The saying "no man is an island" becomes quickly clear to the new dieter who attempts to make his or her emerging hunger pattern mesh with family, business and social schedules. The first few weeks it can seem as if the whole world is in collusion to keep the new 3D dieter from eating at his or her own pace, and Save Your Hungers are a bridge that satisfies the diet's requirements of eating only when at HUNGER LEVEL 3, keeps the dieter from rebelling because of feeling uncomfortably hungry (a major fear of Overeaters), and allows the dieter to continue normal daily patterns of living.

Helpful as they are, we do not recommend that you use Save Your Hungers in the first week of the 3D program because they will interfere with your learning to recognize when you have reached HUNGER LEVEL 3. Experiments have shown that the novice 3D dieter tends to think he or she is at HUNGER LEVEL 3 while still at HUNGER LEVEL 2 or HUNGER LEVEL 2½; so when he uses Save Your Hungers at those levels, it keeps him from losing weight. Now that you are in WEEK TWO of the Dallas Doctors' Diet, however, if you are certain that you can recognize when you reach HUNGER LEVEL 3, you can use Save Your Hungers when necessary.

You will also, of course, continue to:

- eat only at HUNGER LEVEL 3 . . .
- eat anything you want, with the exceptions of cereal, milk, vegetable and fruit juices or sweets, as long as you *taste* your food . . .
- eat in order of preference . . .
- eat slowly for ten minutes, putting your fork down between each bite, and then after the ten minutes are up, stop for five minutes . . .

- take a minimum of twenty minutes to eat each meal . . .
- drink six 10-ounce glasses of water per day . . .
- fill out your Food Sheets.

7

THE
DALLAS DOCTORS'
WEEK TWO

I STUDIED the results of the weekly weigh-in:

Dr. Jerry Bane—down 1 pound
Dr. Cliff Daniel—down 5 pounds
Dr. Mike Mendelson—up ½ pound
Dr. Bill Pirtle—down 1½ pounds
Dr. Sandy Reitman—down 3½ pounds
Dr. Jack Wilson—down 5 pounds

Oh, oh. Doctors Daniel, Reitman and Wilson had done well, but Doctors Bane, Mendelson and Pirtle's Week-Two results had veered from okay to poor.

"Mike, you did so beautifully the first week, losing

eleven pounds, what caused you to *gain* half a pound suddenly?"

"Well, uh . . ."

"Oh, don't misunderstand. I'm not criticizing you, Mike. You look as guilty as if you'd been caught with your hand in the cookie jar."

"Unfortunately that was exactly it. I was doing well, really *well*, when I got sabotaged. I came home, see, and suddenly there was this smell. Carole had baked chocolate chip cookies and when I smelled them I just sort of gravitated toward the kitchen and picked one up. Then another. I'm not a dessert eater, but yeah, I'll eat cookies. But I don't eat *all* cookies. I'm very selective, I'll only eat Carole's chocolate chip cookies or the chocolate cream cookies that come in the package—you know, they've got the cream inside? Not Oreos. Well, Oreos are a big number with me, too, but I wouldn't eat a whole package! Oh, *hell* no. I would just eat a couple. I would eat *four*. I wouldn't eat a package of anything. But I would and did eat all of Carole's homemade ones."

"Well, that certainly would arrest your Fat-Burn-Out mechanism. Every time you eat a dessert it will stop your body's ability to burn off fat for twenty-four hours. Next week I will show you how to satisfy your need for a sweet experience in a way that will allow you to continue to lose weight. Also, Mike, I see on your Food Sheets another reason why you didn't take off any more weight—you forgot on six occasions to take a minimum of twenty minutes per meal.

"Jerry, looking at your Food Sheets, it's amazing that you lost that *one* pound. You ate dessert five times in a row!"

"I wouldn't have, but this was the week of my birthday and I guess I got carried away."

"When you went without breakfast Saturday and Sunday, Jerry, how did you feel?"

"Hungry. I get up pretty early and run and *then* go back and eat breakfast and both days I was at a full HUNGER LEVEL 3, I think. I did do two things right this week, Sandra. You said no to cereal and I'm learning to survive without it. I eat an English muffin or whole wheat toast instead. And water."

"Are you missing your milk a lot?"

"Not really, and I'm flabbergasted. As a kid I drank enormous quantities of milk . . . I didn't know you could start the day without drinking milk . . . and I'm beginning to realize that I was still doing that not because I liked it so much but just from *habit.*"

"From what you tell me, I do believe that you have a three-time-a-day hunger pattern, Jerry, and should keep on eating breakfast. If we can get your sweet eating under control, you will do well on this diet. For example, your Food Sheet for Monday (Figure 8) is a well-balanced one except for the strawberry shortcake. If you had had strawberries without the shortcake part you would have lost weight that day, despite having eaten foods that are traditionally considered fattening, like tuna-fish salad, beans and corn bread.

"Bill, you're very easy to diagnose (Figure 9). A one-and-a-half-pound weight loss is good, but I know you're disappointed not to have done a bit better. I suspect that what did you in was that you ate too fast and so ate too much. The reason I know this is that you took the five-minute breaks only three times this week. Also, Bill, you have a two-time-a-day hunger pattern, yet on Tuesday you slowed down your Fat-Burn-Out mechanism by eating half a grapefruit at eight-thirty in the morning. You

Jerry Bane

TIME OF DAY	LEVEL OF HUNGER	FOOD EATEN AND AMOUNT	TIME TAKEN TO EAT
6:60	*3*	*whole wheat toast*	*5 min.*
12:30	*3*	*tuna-fish salad*	*20 min.*
8:00	*3*	*brown beans* *corn bread* *cherry tomatoes* *strawberry shortcake*	*25 min.*

5 MIN. BREAK + +

WATER + + + + +

Figure 8

marked down that you were at HUNGER LEVEL 3, but
I doubt this. It is more likely that you were at a 1½ or,
at *most*, a 2, else you couldn't have re-reached HUNGER
LEVEL 3 as early as twelve-thirty.

"Let's see, we covered the subject of food myths pretty
well last week. Did any of you succumb to a flirt food?"

"I didn't succumb," Dr. Cliff Daniel said, "but I realized
that hospitals have a booby trap that doctors are always
walking into—those free doughnuts and coffee the auxili-
ary provides."

"Or if there are muffins around. It rarely happened
. . . I'm talking once a month . . . but before you talked
about this flirt food thing, I would take a very small . . .
small! . . . doughnut or whatever was there," Dr. Mike
Mendelson acknowledged.

Dr. Bill Pirtle reported, "I found it hard to resist the
canapés that are always being passed around at parties.
Joyce and I went to a cocktail party and a gallery opening
this week and trays of canapés were always being waved
under my nose. In the past I've tended to munch on
those things mostly for something to do, not because I
was hungry, I now realize."

"Also," Dr. Cliff Daniel remarked, "no one has mentioned that patients bring you foods in the office, which
certainly qualify as flirt foods."

"My wife, Marsha, and daughter Margaret are big chip
eaters," said Dr. Jerry Bane, "and it's easy to just dip a
hand in a bowl of chips without thinking because they're
sitting out on the table or counter."

"Have you become more selective in your food combinations in this past week?" I asked.

"I'll tell you what I've started doing," Dr. Sandy Reitman reported. "I love the skins of baked potatoes. The

Bill Pirtle

TIME OF DAY	LEVEL OF HUNGER	FOOD EATEN AND AMOUNT	TIME TAKEN TO EAT
8:30	3	one-half grapefruit	10 min.
12:30	3	2 fried eggs 3 sausage patties 1 piece buttered toast	20 min.
7:00	3	1 small tenderloin steak 1 cup french fries	35 min.

5 MIN. BREAK   X

WATER X X X X X X

Figure 9

potato inside I can take or leave. So the other night I ordered the butter on the side. Then I scooped out the bulk of the potato onto the plate and ignored it. Then I filled the skin with butter, salt and pepper and just ate that. There's no reason to go through a whole potato just to eat the skins."

Dr. Cliff Daniel said, "I stopped dressing up my potatoes this week. I found I prefer to have 'em blank rather than with butter, sour cream and chives or cheese."

"I'm not sure if this falls under the category of eating too fast or Unthinking Food Combinations," Sandy related, "but before this diet I ate too fast and I now realize that in eating fast you tend to overspice foods. You need that aftertaste that lets you know that a meal passed through. I can wipe out a restaurant-size bottle of Tabasco in a month, one of those great big bottles, and I've even been carrying miniature Tabascos with me to places where I think they might not have any. I've been putting Tabasco on things that don't deserve it because I wolf my food. The pain in my mouth and in my belly told me that I had eaten a meal! But this week, because I'm slowing down, I began really appreciating flavors. Suddenly I could tell that the Tabasco was terrible, that it ruined the subtleties."

Jack Wilson spoke up. "I'll tell you what's nearly blown my mind this week, Sandra, is crackers. I used to never take crackers because they're hard and you have to chew them, but now I love them. I've found that Triscuits are just fantastic. I just love them. I'm eating four or five Triscuits with a little piece of cheese for lunch every day, and it's all I want. I had never *tasted* a cracker until your taste test last week. And I liked that crunch. I *need* that crunch. I have to have it at every meal now, just like you said, or I'm not satisfied. I do think that crunchy foods are generally healthier than soft foods. When you eat most of your soft foods, like the cakes, the goo, the cookies and ice cream, you don't do anything with your teeth. Oh. All of a sudden I'm eating *apples* too, to get that crunch."

"Does anyone think he is a soft food eater?" I asked.

Bill Pirtle replied, "I'm not sure. Can you be both a soft and crunchy eater?"

"Yes, you can, Bill. And some people go through alternating cycles—all soft foods for a while, then all crunchy or chewy foods for a while. It doesn't matter which you like the most as long as you make sure to get whatever texture you need for fiber balance into each meal. Although I do agree with you, Jack, that you need to eat some chewy foods each day for the sake of tooth and gum health.

"I noticed, Cliff, that you're the only one in the group who used Save Your Hungers this week—and you also had one of the highest weight losses."

"I got hungry around three or four o'clock two or three times this week and went across the street and had a teaspoon of peanut butter. It works! I was very surprised that I could look forward to scooping up a teaspoon of peanut butter, but I'm beginning to rely on this pretty heavily. It works best if I take a lot of time with it. If you just take the spoon and pop a little peanut butter in your mouth it's not nearly as effective as if you kinda labor over it a little bit."

"They're handy," Wayne corroborated. "I use them about five or five-thirty because it's six before I ever get out of the office, and if I make rounds, it's seven or eight before I get home. Jerry, with your screwball schedule,

I would think that Save Your Hungers would help you a great deal when you're in a long surgery and reach HUNGER LEVEL 3."

"I intend to use them. I get called in for emergency late-night surgery three or four evenings a week, and then if I happen to be on call on the weekend I can be assured of being called in several times during those days and nights. That's why I don't have a whole lot of sympathy for patients who tell me, 'I'm too busy to lose weight.' It's a cop-out."

"I wish we could get every overweight person who's scheduled for elective surgery on a diet," said Wayne. "It would make their procedures so much easier to do."

"Why is that?" I wanted to know.

Jerry explained, "Fat makes surgery very difficult technically. If you have somebody that's slim and trim, the anatomy's easy. You can see everything. But if they're fat, there's literally flab globbin' everywhere, especially in the abdomen. It's really hard to work."

"I disagree with you, Jerry, that it's more difficult for busy people to diet," Bill Pirtle said. "When you're busy you don't think about eating. It never enters your mind. If you have a three-hour operation or you're busy in the office seeing one patient after another, you never think about food. It's the bored person that has the big handicap, especially the housewife who sends her husband off to work and kids to school and she's stuck doing housework all day. Housework is boring and these women become picky eaters, pick, pick, picking at food all day because they don't have anything to distract them from wanting food."

"It's not just women who work in the home who are prone to overeating. Even the businesswoman, if she is responsible for her family's meal planning, shopping, food preparation and kitchen clean-ups is going to be tempted to eat too much too often because she's constantly encountering flirt food situations the average male doesn't face," I pointed out.

"Also," Wayne said, "women don't lose as many pounds per week as men do. Women normally tend to store more fat on their bodies than men do. Nature just designed women that way."

"Does this mean that women won't do as well on this diet as we're doing?" Jack Wilson asked.

"Not at all. Women tend to lose weight more slowly than men on *any* diet, Jack, but I've found that both men and women get good results on my diet as long as they eat only when hungry, drink the water and control their sugar intake. Which brings me to the point in my course that several of you have been waiting for very impatiently: A Sweet Experience—Week Three of the Dallas Doctors' Diet."

8

WEEK THREE OF THE DALLAS DOCTORS' DIET

I SOMETIMES THINK that Week Three of my diet gives me my nicest feelings as a teacher, because getting to eat sweets again makes many of you so very happy. I don't happen to be much of a sweet eater anymore, but there was a time when I was so in need of Sweet Experiences that if there had been a brick wall between me and a chocolate cake, the brick wall would have lost. So I understand your desire to have a food that means so much to you restored to your dining table.

There are five reasons why I haven't allowed you to eat sweets during the initial stages of the 3D program:

1. Chocolate and sugar foods throw out such power-

134

ful lures that they would have distracted you from your efforts to identify, and then return to, your body's normal hunger patterns.

2. Desserts, more than any other type of food, tend to be eaten at HUNGER LEVEL 2, which, as you now know, would put weight on you.

3. Chocolate and sugar foods can be so addictive that you could be eating them not because you *like* their taste a lot, but because your body has come to crave them. The only way to find out if you are a chocolate or sugar junkie is to free your body of its daily sweet fix long enough to let you experiment with, and savor, regular food flavors and textures.

4. You have needed these two weeks of practice in eating slowly. Studies have shown that Overeaters eat *desserts* faster than any other part of the meal.

5. You have needed awareness of, and practice in, appeasing the satiety center in your hypothalamus with small quantities of the rich foods.

Sugar wasn't a major temptation to our grandparents because there wasn't much of it around. In 1900, the average person in the United States consumed 4 *ounces* of sugar per year. Today, the average person eats 128 *pounds* of sugar per annum. So, since sweets have probably become an almost daily threat/pleasure in your life, you must develop skill to keep sugar in its place.

You want to be master/mistress of your sweet experiences, not a slave, so this week you will learn how to *control* your sugar intake so that you can continue to get that all-important sweet sensation that is necessary to your eating happiness. Control will (1) remove your worries about getting fat; (2) decrease the amount of your sugar intake, thus minimizing your health risk; and (3) stop your secret, furtive, sweet-eating patterns . . . those awful sugar binges that fill you with self-loathing and make your scales jump.

You have become aware in the last two weeks that you can eat a big plate of spaghetti and meat sauce when you're at HUNGER LEVEL 3 and not gain weight. You can't do this with a big plate of cheesecake. I cannot give you a scientific explanation, but I know from my years of working with people with weight problems that eating high sugar content foods such as ice-cream sundaes, candy bars, pies, and cake will literally STOP your Fat-Burn-Out mechanism in its tracks for twenty-four hours. I am not a scientist, so I can only guess why this is so. My suspicion is that there is no element included in your body's enzymes, hormones and cells capable of turning the chemical components of sugar into a fully utilizable food; therefore sugar clogs up your body's usually efficient digestive machinery and it takes a while for your body to clean that clogging residue of sugar out of your system and get itself back to normal fat-efficient functioning.

If you put diesel fuel into a car not designed to utilize that kind of fuel, that car isn't going to run properly until it's rid of the "alien" fuel, right? I suspect that the same is true of your body when you ingest desserts and candy in any quantity.

I also suspect that caloric density is a major factor. Sweets have extremely high caloric density, and I have noticed that the more dense the sugar food the harder it is for your Fat-Burn-Out mechanism to function.

Take a look at the CALORIC DENSITY CHART I have compiled (Figure 10) and you will get a picture of what

CALORIC DENSITY OF SWEETS

Sugar products can both interfere with and stop your body's natural ability to burn fat.

*   *   *

1 slice of Crisco icing birthday = 6 large bananas
  cake with scoop of ice cream   or

  1 pound of fried onion rings
               or
  2 chicken pot pies
               or
  7 crescent dinner rolls
               or
  1 Big Mac hamburger with or-
    der of fries
               or
  2 baked potatoes with 4 T. but-
    ter & sour cream
               or
  ¾ pound of cooked pot roast

1 slice of homemade pecan pie = a 10-ounce slice of ham
               or
  4½ English muffins (whole)
               or
  9½ slices of whole wheat
    bread
               or
  33 Ritz crackers
               or
  65 Wheat Thins
               or
  6 large pears

Figure 10

CALORIC DENSITY OF SWEETS (*Continued*)

1 package of M&M's = 1 sourdough French roll with 2
pats butter
or
6 large peaches

1 Snickers bar of candy = 1 chocolate éclair
or
large corn on the cob with 2
T. butter
or
9 small pancakes
or
10 cups raw cauliflower buds
or
28 Melba Toast Rounds

2 small slices chocolate cake = 4½ pounds of raw carrots
or
4 12-ounce beers
or
a 10-ounce sirloin strip steak
or
2 Burger King chocolate milk
shakes

Cheesecake . . . average = 1 omelet with bacon
serving
or
80 almonds
or
40 cups of chicken bouillon
or
3 shrimp eggrolls

CALORIC DENSITY OF SWEETS (*Continued*)

                              or
                              1 pound of cooked red beans
                              or
                              1½ slices of sausage pizza

1 slice of banana cream pie   = 3 cups of apple cider
                              or
                              an 8-ounce bowl of chili
                              or
                              70 stalks of celery
                              or
                              5 slices of raisin bread
                              or
                              20 apricots
                              or
                              1 bag of crunchy Cheetos with dip

4 chocolate chip cookies   = 4 Popsicles
(homemade)
                              or
                              3 cups of papaya
                              or
                              80 spears of asparagus
                              or
                              5 cups of puffed rice cereal
                              or
                              2 8-ounce glasses of orange juice
                              or
                              ¼ of a pound of corned beef
                              or
                              24 medium oysters

CALORIC DENSITY OF SWEETS (*Continued*)

2 scoops pralines and cream = 22 cups boiled zucchini
ice cream

or

8 ounces of tuna salad

or

1 pound of lemon yogurt

or

8 cups of watermelon

or

1 pound of sole

or

8 small link pork sausages

or

4 pounds of fresh tomatoes

I'm talking about. For example, a 2-*ounce* chocolate bar has the same caloric density as three medium-size bananas, which would weigh approximately *a full pound!* One slice of birthday cake with a single scoop of ice cream is the equivalent of 7 pounds of honey dew melon, and one piece of pecan pie is the equal of 65 Wheat Thins!!

Now I'm not trying to discourage you from eating sweets. If you love them, I hope you go ahead and enjoy sugar foods so that you won't suffer any feelings of frustration or deprivation. If you follow my instructions on HOW to eat desserts, you will be able to minimize their fattening character. After all, True Thins eat desserts without gaining weight, so you can too, if you eat them in the same fashion.

Let's start your Sweet Experience with almost everyone's favorite candy—chocolate. Put three squares of a Hershey chocolate bar and a quarter of a Fun-Size Baby Snickers bar on a taster plate.

Hershey bar. Pick up one square of chocolate and chew it up as fast as you can. This is the way most Overeaters (that used to be you, remember?) consume chocolate. People with a weight problem feel so much guilt about eating sweets that a chocolate bar is generally wolfed down and the wrapper thrown in the waste paper basket in under three minutes! After today I doubt that you will eat chocolate that way.

Pick up the second square of chocolate and put it in your mouth. If any chocolate has stuck to your fingers, lick it off. Now give the chocolate a minute to warm up so that it will start to melt, then gently move it to your left cheek, then to your right cheek. Next, rub it over your teeth. You are playing with chocolate in the same way children do. They don't overeat on chocolate because they instinctively know how to get the most enjoyment out of it.

Now take the third piece of chocolate and place it on your tongue. Again, let it warm up. Then slide it under your tongue. Play with this piece entirely with your tongue, letting it get coated with the velvety, buttery morsel until your taste buds become satiated with chocolate, chocolate, chocolate. Do you enjoy it more when you get the full texture and taste of the chocolate? Do you like *not* chewing it?

Snickers. Take your quarter of a piece of Fun-Size Snickers bar and place it in your mouth. Don't bite down on it. Let the chocolate slowly melt, then chew the caramel layer, and lastly, crunch on the peanuts. You will notice that a Snickers will give you three separate sensuous sensations when you eat it this way—melt, chew and crunch. How do you like America's number-one-selling candy bar? An Overeater would probably have eaten a whole, regular-size, 1¾-ounce Snickers bar in the time you took to eat your tiny piece, but I'm willing to bet that you got more taste and pleasure out of your sliver of Snickers than Overeaters do with the whole bar. By the way, if you study your CALORIC DENSITY CHART, you will see that eating a full-size Snickers bar would be the equivalent food density experience of gobbling up about a pound of apples in three minutes! A most unsatisfactory way of enjoying food, wouldn't you agree?

There are several "tricks" that you can use to aid your controlling quantity when you want a sweet experience:

1. Eat a raw carrot before the sweet. Your fullness center will register more quickly and help keep you from overeating.

2. Eat all desserts v-e-r-y, v-e-r-y slowly. A piece of pie or cake should take twenty minutes to eat.

3. Refrigerate your chocolate bar for a short time before eating it. This will make the chocolate melt more slowly and stretch the time and pleasure of your Sweet Experience.

4. If you crave a dessert but don't know what, choose an ice-cream cone, because licking takes much longer than spooning.

5. Look up the dessert of your choice on the CALORIC DENSITY CHART before eating it and then keep the comparison in mind when ingesting it. While you're eating a slice of chocolate cake, for example, take as long to finish it as it would take you to ingest its counterpart— four beers!

You can achieve your Sweet Experience this week in one of two ways. The first is to use a sweet as a closure to a meal. Some people feel the need of a "little something sweet" to finish a meal, but don't want or need a whole dessert to be happy. If this is your pattern, then you can have any sweet "finisher" of your choice this week at dinner as long as that finisher does not exceed 50 calories. Take a look at A SWEET EXPERIENCE AS A CLOSURE CHART (Figure 11) to see how to use sweets as a closure.

Notice that little box beside the finisher? This week I want you to draw a square on your Food Sheet beside any sweet you eat and enter the number of calories in the box. My SUGAR CALORIE COUNTER (Figure 12) will help you figure the correct number of calories.

A SWEET EXPERIENCE AS A CLOSURE CHART

TIME OF DAY	LEVEL OF HUNGER	FOOD EATEN AND AMOUNT	TIME TAKEN TO EAT
1:00	3	1 fish fillet mixed fruit 2 corn fritters	25 min.
7:30	3	2 pieces of fried chicken 6 french fries 2 bites apple pie 50	35 min.
		5 MIN. BREAK ✓ ✓ WATER ✓ ✓ ✓ ✓ ✓ ✓	

Figure 11

MY SUGAR CALORIE COUNTER

CANDY

1 Kiss	28*	1 Kraft Fudgie	35
1 Kraft caramel	33	1 jelly bean	12
1 Coffee Nip	26	1 choc. cov. cherry	66
1 butterscotch	17	1 peppermint pattie	109
1 malted milk ball	9	1 choc. cov. peanut	12
1 Baby Snickers	90	1 oz. M&M	140
1 Hershey bar	180	1 reg. Snickers	240
1 peanut butter cup	224	1 Milky Way	220
1 toffee bar	206	1 oz. peanut brittle	132

PIES

1 avg. piece pecan	585*	⅙ chocolate meringue	353
⅙ strawberry	356	⅙ chocolate chiffon	459
⅙ homemade apple	404	⅙ homemade peach	403
⅙ cherry	412	⅙ lemon ice box	438

JELLIES, PRESERVES AND SYRUPS

1 T. apple	52*	1 T. honey	61
1 T. cherry	53	1 T. syrup	50
1 T. grape	54	1 tsp. Thick Syrup	70
1 tsp. jam	19	1 tsp. preserves	20

JUICES

½ cup apple juice	70*	½ cup prune juice	92
½ cup cranberry juice	83	½ cup orange juice	59
½ cup unsweetened pineapple	74	½ cup grape juice	84
½ cup grapefruit	48	½ cup sweetened pineapple juice	90

* Figures are equivalent to calorie counts for amounts stated.

Figure 12

YOGURTS

½ 8-oz. carton plain ... 76*
½ 8-oz. carton coffee .. 100
½ 8-oz. carton cherry .. 184
½ 8-oz. carton peach .. 149

½ 8-oz. carton
   pineapple 152
1 cone frozen yogurt 250

MILK PRODUCTS

1 8-oz. chocolate milk .. 212*
1 8-oz. plain milk 151

1 small McDonald's
   chocolate shake 363
   vanilla 347
   strawberry 322

DOUGHNUTS

1 sm. cake type 125*
1 choc. covered 280
1 glazed 254

1 chocolate eclair 325
1 sweet roll with nuts
   and icing............ 325

COOKIES

1 choc. chip 52–80*
1 cinnamon 13–17
1 coconut 47–80
1 Pecan Sandy 85
1 Oreo 51

1 fig bar 45–71
1 gingersnap 24–30
1 oatmeal 70–80
1 Vanilla Wafer 15–20

CAKE

cheesecake ⅙ of
   8″ cake 483*

angel food 1/12 of
   8″ cake.............. 108

* Figures are equivalent to calorie counts for amounts stated.

CAKE

chocolate ¹⁄₁₂ of
  9″ cake 365

coffee cake ⅛ 181

avg. banana pudding
  serving 336

ICE CREAM

1 scoop vanilla 250*

1 scoop pralines 275

1 ice cream sandwich .. 208

1 cone . . . only 19

1 choc. coated
  ice cream bar 185

COLD DRINKS

Coke, 6-oz. 73*

Hawaiian Punch, 6-oz. ... 83

Pepsi, 6-oz. 79

CEREALS

Natural . . . Heartland
  and Quaker . . .
  ¼ cup 134
  (with raisins etc.
  add 15 cal.)

Grape Nuts
  (without sugar) . . .
  ¼ cup 100

While on the DALLAS DOCTORS' DIET regard any cereal as a sweet and use calorie counter.

* Figures are equivalent to calorie counts for amounts stated.

If your heart's desire is to eat a *whole* dessert this week, you may do so ONCE. The dessert chosen must not exceed 500 calories, and *this dessert should take the place of other food.* This is called A FULL SWEET EXPERIENCE. See the Food Sheet in Figure 13 for the correct way of adding this delightful taste bonanza to your diet.

I suspect you are thinking, "Sandra, you aren't being overly generous in your sugar allowance." But what other

A FULL SWEET EXPERIENCE

TIME OF DAY	LEVEL OF HUNGER	FOOD EATEN AND AMOUNT	TIME TAKEN TO EAT
1:00 p.m.	*3*	*Greek salad crackers pear*	*35 min.*
6:30 p.m.	*3*	*1 piece of chocolate cake*	*20 min.*

400

NOTE: You may follow the cake with a very little food, such as a bite or two of cheese, a bite of hamburger or a few peanuts. These foods then become the closure of your meal.

5 MIN. BREAK √ √
WATER √ √ √ √ √ √

Figure 13

diet allows you to eat ANY sweets?! And on what other diet could you eat sweets and *not* gain all your hard-lost weight back? And what other diet gives you the tools to tame your sugar monster, and keep that monster subdued for the rest of your life? On my diet you can have your cake and eat it too. The fact that you are eating less will not matter to you as you become aware that by eating it in this new True Thin way you are enjoying it more!

DR. WAYNE AGNEW'S CAPSULE COMMENTS:

You have been given "permission" to add sweets to your diet this week, and if you desire them, by all means go ahead and enjoy them. Do keep in mind, however, that that piece of coconut cream pie or butterscotch parfait will stop your Fat-Burn-Out for twenty-four hours and, obviously, slow down your weight loss this week. I remind you of this not to dissuade you from a Sweet Experience, but to keep you from being disappointed if you don't achieve as high a weight loss as in the preceding week. A fine dessert can be well worth a day's delay in weight reduction. The point is that the decision is yours. You are in control and you're not a bad person if you eat the dessert and a good person if you don't. The correct decision should be based on what will best meet your needs this week.

One word of warning: If you do eat a dessert, be sure you *don't* have alcohol during the same twenty-four hours, because alcohol and sugar combined increase the length of time your Fat-Burn-Out mechanism will be unable to attend to its primary duty of getting you thin. A patient of mine dubbed the effects of mixing alcohol and sugar "The Double Whammy," and I consider the nickname appropriate.

When you do eat sweets this week, remember that you can choose only *one* of the two styles, either:

- 50 calories per day as closure (A SWEET EXPERIENCE AS A CLOSURE),

or

- 500 calories once a week (A FULL SWEET EXPERIENCE).

9
THE DALLAS DOCTORS' WEEK THREE

THE DALLAS DOCTORS' Week Three weigh-in figures looked very good:

Dr. Jerry Bane—2 pounds
Dr. Cliff Daniel—4 pounds
Dr. Mike Mendelson—3¼ pounds
Dr. Bill Pirtle—4 pounds
Dr. Sandy Reitman—4¼ pounds
Dr. Jack Wilson—4½ pounds

"What a truly outstanding job you've done this week," I told the Dallas Doctors. "I can't praise you enough. Does anyone still find it difficult to distinguish HUNGER LEVEL 3 from the other hunger levels?"

Everyone shook his head: no.

"Good. How are you doing on drinking your six ten-ounce glasses of water a day?"

Dr. Cliff Daniel reported, "I'm still having trouble with the water. I know I tend to eat more when I don't drink the water, but often I'll have a cup of coffee instead. I've bought myself a good-looking carafe which I've put on my desk so that I'm only an arm's length away from my ice water. I find that this helps. But frankly, it still strikes me as a lot of water. Well, it *is* a lot of water!"

"I've gotten a carafe for my desk, too, Cliff," Dr. Mike Mendelson said. "I wouldn't get up and go get a glass of water. I would have to be very thirsty to do that. But if it's right there on the desk I'll pour a little into a glass and sip it. I'm a sipper. I take a little sip, and then I'll talk to the patients, and then I'll sip some more. But it's taking me time to drink more and more water. I'm not drinking sixty ounces every day yet, maybe forty. Some days fifty. I'd say at *best* I'm drinking sixty ounces of water one day a week. But when you consider that before this diet the most water I'd take in my mouth every day was when I was brushing my teeth, I've come a long way. I'm much more introduced to it then I was before."

Dr. Jack Wilson contributed, "I sip sometimes, but usually I just turn the glass up and drink it. All this water is a hassle, but I drink it anyway. I don't know about anyone else here, but for the first two weeks I couldn't pass a bathroom. But now I can, because I'm learning to manage the water better."

"What are you doing, Jack?" Bill Pirtle wanted to know.

"Well, I usually get up thirsty; in fact I'm so thirsty I try to drink water out of the shower spray! That's pretty thirsty! Then I drink at least ten ounces before going to work. I always try to take another glassful about mid-morning—say ten-thirty—and before every meal I drink a big glass of water. I drink some more water after running in the evening and if I can get it down, a last glass before going to bed."

"I'm finding that it's helpful to make sure that water is always nearby," Bill Pirtle said. "I have about three glasses of water in different places in my office that are kept filled for me, and, of course, at home Joyce makes sure that there is always a big glass of water on the table for me at each meal. I've always drunk a lot of diet drinks, but now I'm not drinking them at all. I drink water and find I prefer it."

"Sandy, you're still only drinking two or three glasses of water a day. That's not enough."

"I know, I know. But look, I don't drink a lot of liquids normally. Truly I don't, although I appreciate that they're important for normal health. I'm just not able to get the water down. I don't *dislike* water; I like sailing, I'm a swimmer of sorts. Maybe I had a bad experience in the intrauterine life or something, I can't explain it.

"Since you're something of a gourmet, Sandy, perhaps you could try drinking a bottled or carbonated water."

"I don't think it's the flavor that's keeping me from drinking the water. I've tried carbonated water, plain ordinary soda water, fancy mineral waters. At the airport the other night I asked for a Perrier at one of those little airport bars, and the bartender said, 'We don't have any, we just have plain club soda,' and I was *thrilled*, because I think Perrier is terrible. Not enough carbonation in it. I have distilled water at home, but I don't drink that either except in tea. I'm willing to do everything else on your diet, but I just can't drink as much water as you say I should."

"I've never had anyone in a class with a block against water like you have, Sandy. We'll just have to work around your antipathy. Can you bring yourself to drink more iced tea throughout the day and perhaps let the ice in the tea melt enough to dilute the tea and add to your liquid volume? This way you will continue to keep your body cells hydrated enough so Fat-Burn-Out can take place. You won't lose as *much* weight per week with the iced tea, but you will lose some."

"I'll give it a try. I'm already doing what you suggested to some extent, and it seems to be pretty effective."

"Jerry, your Achilles heel is desserts, but you must have handled them better this week because you doubled your weight-loss figure of last week."

"I've cut back because I discovered that if I eat something sweet like candy, it almost invariably gives me a headache an hour or two later. Shortly after that I feel shaky and really hungry. If I don't eat anything, the hunger passes in a relatively short time, but if I eat something sweet and don't eat later, I feel shaky."

"Do you get shaky and headachy when you eat other foods?"

"No, only desserts and candy. But I'm not willing to give them up. What I did this week was cut down the quantities by eating sugar closures most nights and full desserts two times. Now I know that isn't ideal, but two desserts per week is a big improvement over seven per week. The SWEETS AS A CLOSURE is helping me control my sweet tooth. I think I'll always have a problem with sweets, but finding I can cut my sugar intake by about one-half is gratifying."

"You may find after awhile that you do even better, Jerry," Cliff said. "I always felt that no meal was complete without some kind of dessert, but because of the new ways I'm eating on this diet, I've lost my desire for sugar. My favorite dessert is apple pie. I have something of a reputation in our family for the amount of apple pie I can put away. We had an apple tree in our backyard in Maryland and my mother-in-law would bake pies as fast as I could eat them. I must have eaten about thirty apple pies one month. *Huge* apple pies. But the point of all this is that this week, when I had the opportunity to eat apple pie again, I didn't take it. I didn't feel hungry for dessert and I'm doing so well I didn't want to risk triggering a desire for sweets again."

"Also, knowing that you can have that dessert any time you want it helps you put off going for it," Jack Wilson said. "Sugar is my worst enemy. Look. I'm all gold. Inlays, onlays, crowns, whatever. That's from sugar. Sugar's bad. There's no nutritional value to sugar. Not any. But you always hear that sugar's a pick-me-up. 'Gonna get me a little quick energy. Gonna get me some sugar.' I have one patient, a girl, who drinks three family-size bottles of coke a day and *adds* sugar to them. I was never *that* bad."

"How did you handle your sugar problem this week, Jack?"

"Before this diet, every night I would run until eight or nine and then come in and have my three to six dips of praline ice cream, so I thought that's what I'd probably do this week—except fewer dips. But now here's what surprised me. After being off sugar for two weeks I didn't really want it, so I didn't eat *any* this week. If you'd told me a month ago that I could go three weeks without cookies or ice cream or *something* sweet, I'd have just laughed at you."

"Mike, did you eat any desserts this week?"

"No. After eating all those cookies last week I just made up my mind I better lay off for awhile and I did."

"Sandy, you aren't a sweet eater, so I'll pass you by. Bill?"

"I used the SWEETS AS A CLOSURE technique and found it worked very well. For instance, one night I had three bites of chocolate cake, another night four bites of Jello fruit salad, and another evening two small bites of lemon chess pie. On those nights that I had a couple of Scotch and waters before dinner, I didn't finish the meal with a sweet closure."

"Excellent. Did everyone take their five-minute breaks?"

"Now *that* is hard," Dr. Bill Pirtle admitted. "I always take at least twenty to twenty-five minutes to eat, but I don't take a true five-minute break. I take several one minute breaks. I'll open my mail maybe or read the paper. Is that all right?"

"It's unusual, but I can tell it's working for you, Bill, because you're taking enough time overall to eat and your quantities of food are down."

Dr. Cliff Daniel said, "I keep having trouble remembering to take the five-minute break. I actually took out my watch and timed myself in the beginning. I am slowing down some. I always used to finish dinner faster than my wife, even though she ate less food, but now we're finishing at nearly the same time."

Dr. Jerry Bane commented, "I think the real secret of this diet is the eating slowly and learning to be sensitive to when you are satisfied. When I do that I just don't need as much food. Also, I feel the water is important."

"I agree, Jerry," Mike Mendelson said. "Before this program I was a *fast* eater. I mean I would eat so fast that sometimes I wouldn't even chew. I would gulp food."

"I saw that, Mike. Why, last week you ate a whole dinner in *four* minutes. You are the fastest eater I've ever had in my course. But during Week One you did beautifully, and this week you have a perfect record. You took the five-minute break and apparently ate each bite slowly. I think we can change you from a hare into a tortoise."

"That could be. This week I got the feeling that eating slowly could be something I could adjust to."

"One thing puzzles me on your Food Sheets, Mike. You ate the same main course for dinner Monday through Wednesday and then on Thursday and Friday you again had identical dinners. I'm worried that you're not getting enough variety in your diet—that you're not indulging your food preferences."

"Yeah, I sorta noticed that, too. What happened was that Carole is so used to making big, I mean *big* amounts of food for me that she didn't know how to cut back on quantity and so, since I'm eating so much less, we had all these leftovers. Leftovers are something very new in our house. So I just ate what was there each night when I got home. We're getting this problem solved."

Sandy spoke up. "I'm finding that if I stop for five minutes as you directed, and allow myself that time lapse for the 'full' message to arrive from my belly, by George, I actually *am* full! I can't tell you how many times in the past I've gotten up from the table and said, 'I ate too much!' No more. Jerry, you feel the secret of this diet is eating slowly and drinking the water. The secret for me is simply being able to identify when I am hungry (HUNGER LEVEL 3) and when I am full, although unquestionably, in learning to eat slowly my enjoyment of food has improved considerably. We used to eat beef twenty-nine days a month, poultry maybe once. And I have always refused to eat fish. Never cared for it. But this is changing. We ate beef three times this week and fish and poultry the rest of the time. I have no idea why, but in learning to eat slowly I am starting to enjoy some of the seafood flavors more than I did."

"Do you have any criticism of the diet now that you have been on it for twenty-one days?" I wanted to know. "Please be frank."

"Only what I said before," Jack Wilson commented, "that drinking that much water makes you have to go to the bathroom a lot and it took me awhile to figure out how to space each glass of water so that I wasn't always having to excuse myself suddenly from what I was doing."

"I think most people would have a hard time in the beginning telling the difference between appetite and hunger," Cliff Daniel said. "We're all doctors and *we* still went through a little trial and error."

"Some dieters could feel panicky if they misjudged their hunger level, and ended up at HUNGER LEVEL 4 before they ate," Mike Mendelson pointed out. "People who are food-dependent aren't used to deferring oral gratification so they might have some trouble dealing with this diet in the first week . . . especially if they leaned pretty heavily on snacking to get them through daily stresses in the past."

Sandy spoke out. "But in all fairness, this diet is a picnic compared to standard reducing regimens. My wife, Margaret, will tell you that in the twenty-five years we've been married I've been on a diet at least once a year and every time I've been a totally miserable person and made my whole family miserable too. When I can't eat what I want, I feel deprived, and there's no way you can console me short of giving me back those foods I want. Margaret told me after the first week on your diet, Sandra, that this time I'm just like a different person. This has made my wife very happy. I have changed my eating habits drastically, and yet Margaret was able to cook the same meals every day that she normally cooks, and it was just miraculous the way neither she nor my family or friends were aware when they've eaten with me that I'm on a special food program. This is the first time in my whole life that I've experienced what it's like to eat and feel like what you call a True Thin. I'm not going back to the old deprivation diets."

DR. WAYNE AGNEW'S CAPSULE COMMENTS:

The Dallas Doctors' total weight losses for the first three weeks on the 3D diet are most impressive:

Dr. Jerry Bane—8 pounds
Dr. Cliff Daniel—13 pounds
Dr. Mike Mendelson—13¾ pounds
Dr. Bill Pirtle—12 pounds
Dr. Sandy Reitman—13 pounds
Dr. Jack Wilson—17 pounds

The foods the six doctors ate while achieving these impressive weight losses were, by ordinary dieting standards, astounding—lobster, homemade bread, yeast rolls, strawberry shortcake, fried chicken, cheeseburgers, spaghetti, nachos, filet mignon, martinis, blackeyed peas, lasagna, corn on the cob, fried eggs and sausages, chicken salad, tournedos in Madeira sauce, enchiladas, chocolate chip cookies, birthday cake, ice cream, corn bread, glazed ham, chicken Tetrazzini—the list goes on and on.

You can emulate the doctors and eat your favorite foods while you are on the Dallas Doctors' Diet program, but remember that you must not veer away from the precepts of this diet or you will not lose weight, you will gain. The 3D program gives you a license to enter the normal weight world, but if you carry your overweight habits and thinking with you, you will fail in your efforts to be a True Thin.

You are used to forcing preconceived ideas and emotional needs on to your ways of eating. True Thins don't do that. So I recommend that you be on guard during the first few weeks of the 3D program and not let the excess baggage of your fat past interfere with your new food freedom and goals.

Several of the doctors, as you saw, slowed down their weight losses temporarily when they failed to eat only when hungry, when they didn't drink enough water each day and when they overdid on desserts. When you are more experienced at managing the 3D diet, you will be able to "cheat" periodically and not pay the price. But while you are LEARNING the precious skills that will turn you into a True Thin, please follow the few simple rules faithfully. You will be rewarded by steady weight losses, plus a feeling of well-being that you have never known on the usual spartan, punitive diets.

If you have been following the rules of the 3D diet, you should have achieved weight-loss figures that are as gratifying to you as the Dallas Doctors' are to them. Doctors Bane, Daniel, Mendelson, Pirtle, Reitman and Wilson have proved that you can eat your favorite foods and lose weight while doing so. They have shown you that on the 3D diet you can make major changes in your food eating habits without suffering psychologically and emotionally. This is because the changes are happy ones—the banishment of clock-dictated eating and rigid societal rules and the reinstitution of the natural, uniquely individual eating patterns that your body has longed for.

You now have the necessary eating skills to become a True Thin for the rest of your life. If you continue to use these new skills, you will be rewarded with permanent weight losses.

10

WEEK FOUR OF THE DALLAS DOCTORS' DIET

IF YOU ARE typical of most people who take the Naturally Slim course, you will feel impatient about this week's subject. "Just give me the diet instructions," I usually hear, "I'm not interested in examining any of the emotional or psychological reasons why I've become fat."

But after they've completed the program, nearly everyone has said, "You know, Sandra, I resisted the material at the time, but I think Week Four was the second most important week of the course." (Week One was considered the *most* important.)

I am not going to talk about possible major stresses in your life that might send you hurtling toward the comforts of overeating. Marital, job, health, financial and family problems are not in my bailiwick. However, if you are under stress at this time, you can do a great deal to ease your tensions, unhappiness and resorting to overeating for solace by making sure that your special *Vital Needs* are met.

Everyone has Vital Needs—needs that must be satisfied to have a sense of well-being. What do Vital Needs have to do with overeating? If you don't achieve your Vital Needs most of the time you are likely to indulge in binge eating and/or daily eating to excess in a vain attempt to fill the void in you that exists because of those unmet needs.

Oddly enough, many intelligent people are so unaware of the fact that they have Vital Needs that they would find it almost impossible to name even *one* personal need that must be satisfied at least part of the time for them to feel contented. I'd like you to take a look at my VITAL NEEDS SUGGESTION LIST (Figure 14) to see if you recognize any of your personal needs.

VITAL NEEDS SUGGESTION LIST

1. Time Alone. Time for reflection, time for thought.

2. Movement. Shopping, walking, exercise.

3. Sleep. Your day does not go right unless you have a certain amount of sleep.

4. Territory. Physical space. An area that is your very own at home.

5. Anticipation. Something interesting to look forward to each day.

6. A Hobby. A pastime of your choosing.

7. Social Activity. Time spent with companionable people.

   8. **Reading Time.**

   9. **Time to Listen to Music.**

   10. **Opportunity to Give and Do for Others.** Family, community, church.

   11. **Structured Time.** A need for a daily schedule or routine to follow. A need for predictability.

   12. *Un*structured Time. Freedom from following set routines or meeting schedules set by others.

   13. **Sex.**

   14. **Time to Learn Something New.** Information or a skill.

   15. **A Daily Pleasurable Food Experience.**

   16. **Touching.** Physical contact with others.

   17. **Appreciation and Acceptance from Family and Friends.**

   18. **One-on-One Attention.**

   19. **Distance.** Feeling smothered in "togetherness" situations.

   20. **Empathy.** High need for people important to you, or people around you, to know what you are feeling.

   21. **Everything in Its Place.** Tidy surroundings, predictable behavior by loved ones.

   22. **Closure.** A need to complete some projects, tasks or activity daily.

Figure 14

   A number of *my* Vital Needs are on this list. For example, I must have some time alone for reflection; it's important to me to know, when I wake up each day, that I will have something interesting to look forward to; time to read one or more books per week is very important to me; I need the weekly stimulation and excitement of learning a new skill or discovering some new fact; I make sure that I have a *daily* pleasurable food experience; I need to give and do for my family and people I care about and receive their appreciation and attention; and I need closure, the knowledge that at least a few projects, tasks or activities have been "closed out," completed, by the end of each day.

All of my Vital Needs are achievable without too much difficulty most of the time. Yours are too. I make sure that some of my Vital Needs are met *every* day, the rest with some regularity. You can, and have the RIGHT, to do this also. It is not selfish of you to set aside a small island of time and/or emotional energy for activity or contact that nurtures you. Without such nurturing we become less than we can and should be. We shortchange ourselves and those we love because if we are frustrated and unhappy, others find us disappointing to be with. This, obviously, puts strains on relationships.

You can even, if you are pressed for time, pair some Vital Needs. If time alone for thought, exercise, and distance from togetherness are important to you, you can take a brisk walk alone after dinner. You can have a daily pleasurable food experience while listening to music. Touching and sex are natural pair-ups. Social activity and a hobby can be intertwined.

What's important is that you become consciously aware of your particular Vital Needs and then make sure that you never let more than a few days go by without having these needs met. If you do, you will be tempted to overeat as consolation for your frustration.

Dr. Jack Wilson commented, "Basically, I do what I want to do. I already meet my Vital Needs. I have a real need to exercise. I have to do something every day, even if I'm just outside shoveling dirt. My wife realizes I have to exercise. That's how I work out all my frustrations. I also enjoy sports and kids, so I solve that Vital Need by coaching a lot of teams."

"But what have you done in the past, Jack, when you couldn't run or engage in outdoor activities, maybe because you were sick or had to travel or whatever?"

"Now that you mention it, for awhile there I was running five miles a day, but then the weather got bad and I started eating more and running less, like about ten miles a week instead of thirty or forty. Are you suggesting that we be aware of the fact that we should have a *number* of Vital Needs, so that if one can't get met you have others to fall back on to feel good?"

"Exactly, and you should make an effort to balance people-dependent Vital Needs with those you can do alone. For example, if your Vital Needs were:

1. Appreciation
2. Touching
3. Social activity
4. A pleasurable food experience
5. Playing bridge
6. Going fishing

you would be heavily dependent on other people. But people are not always available exactly when you want them to be, so what will you be most likely to do? You will depend too heavily on number four, a pleasurable eating experience, and overeat. The person with the six Vital Needs listed above could study books on advanced bridge techniques when a game is not possible. He might repair his fishing equipment or study catalogs of lures and other paraphernalia. He could develop a solo hobby such as carpentry or gardening. You get the idea. If you are getting a variety of needs met most of the time, you will be less prone to emotionally driven food binges.

"My VITAL NEEDS SUGGESTION LIST is just that—a suggestion list. All of your Vital Needs may be on it, maybe none. Please write out your own list and then make sure that those needs get met regularly.

"You cannot ignore the fact that because you have been Overeaters for so long, any change in your emotional state can lead you to binge on food. Each of you marked on YOUR EATING PROFILE that you ate when you were in both good and bad emotional situations—depressed, nervous, angry, anxious, excited, scared, happy, etc.

"Now you know why eating when you are not hungry will put weight on you, so what should you do when you're confronted with a desire for food? DISTRACT YOURSELF BY MEETING ONE OF YOUR VITAL NEEDS!

"Let's use you, Jerry, as an example. You run every morning about six, but let's assume that you get called in at four in the morning to do emergency surgery. You get finished at six-thirty, too late to go back home and run, too early to start your rounds. Instead of making a bee-line for the cafeteria and those tempting sweet rolls, pancakes or waffles, how about sitting down in your office for twenty minutes while you have this rare quiet moment and reading the latest issue of the ski magazine you subscribe to but seldom get time to enjoy? Or if you need a more energetic activity, run around the block or walk up and then back down several flights of stairs, or put a mini-trampoline in your office and bounce up and down for a few minutes.

"Walk away from, or distract yourself with, activities

other than eating when you are in emotional situations that make you want to reach for food. Bill, you're an art collector. If you have a stressful morning and maybe an unhappy one because of having to give bad news to a patient or two, don't eat; get out of your office for half an hour and take a quick tour of an art gallery. You will find that this will please you emotionally and intellectually much more than eating a piece of pie you're not hungry for."

Dr. Mike Mendelson spoke. "There's no question that a tremendous amount of stress is focused in people's eating habits. It's very interesting to see how our daily frustrations interact with the way we eat. I've been thinking, while you've been talking about feelings and Vital Needs, that you've explained to me why I eat so much at social functions. You see, I'm a very shy person. It's *true*. You're laughing, but it's true. For me, eating is a way of not having to talk, of not having to deal with people at a social level. For instance, I'm going to a banquet tomorrow night. You know what's going to happen? All I'm gonna do all night is meet people. I'm going to go, 'Oh, God, I don't know who this guy is. Gimme the shrimp. Where's the shrimp? I'll get lost in the shrimp bowl for awhile. Then, 'Oh, God, I don't wanna talk to that guy, so I'll run over to the fruit bowl. If I have to talk to somebody, it'll be, 'God, did you see the shrimp bowl someplace? Where's that? Is it over there? Thank you!' But how can I change this? I'm a shy person, and I doubt that I'm going to change that and become some kind of a glad-hander extrovert."

"When Carole can't go with you to banquets, make sure that you go with a colleague you like to talk to and stick with him," Dr. Cliff Daniel suggested.

"Or you could arrive late . . . after all the cocktail-type food has been served," said Dr. Jerry Bane.

"Or you can make sure you're one of the speakers. Speakers *never* get to eat at these affairs," laughed Dr. Jack Wilson.

"I'm serious," Mike Mendelson protested. "I eat emotionally. Awhile back, for instance, I was very bad. I was getting out of group and into private practice, and I was feeling kind of blue. I didn't know if it was the right thing to do; I had a lot of questions. So what I would do is, when there was a break, if I didn't have any consults or I was finished up, I'd go over to the hospital cafeteria and eat. Somehow, I don't know how, I *made* that happen."

"But now that you have some insight into the fact that you eat around feelings, Mike, you can distract yourself by meeting one of your Vital Needs. Pick up the phone and talk to your kids. Write your wife a note about what you're worried or happy about at the moment. Play a video game if you enjoy that. Do the *New York Times* crossword puzzle. Anything that gives you pleasure will do. The key, as I'm sure you're all beginning to realize, is to know what your Vital Needs are, and then which ones can be filled in office or short time-span situations. I always have an exciting book with me. I sometimes will call my husband Justin up and tell him I love him and am thinking of him. The telephone, when you make a pleasurable personal call, can be a very useful device. Morley Safer, the famous co-host of TV's *60 Minutes*, sketches or paints the boring hotel rooms he has to spend so much time in, and he does it so well he recently had an exhibition of his hotel-room paintings at a major New York art gallery."

Most women can tick off at least five Vital Needs without even having to give it much thought; the average man needs time to think about what is important to him on a daily and weekly basis. So your assignment for Week Four is:

1. Make a list of at least five Vital Needs, and
2. Meet each of these Vital Needs at least once during this week.

DR. WAYNE AGNEW'S CAPSULE COMMENTS:

If you have a longtime pattern of eating around feelings, then knowledge of your Vital Needs is critical to your future success in keeping your weight off.

Understanding the importance of Vital Needs has helped me considerably. It used to be that when I got disgusted and angry I would reach for food. Now I don't do that because a little light goes on in my head to warn me that eating isn't going to make my anger or frustration go away. Then I think what *would* make me feel better, and I go and do that.

I don't think the fact that I was unaware that I have Vital Needs is unusual. It's been my experience as a doctor that women don't mind exploring their feelings, but, historically, men don't talk a whole lot about emotions and needs. When I was growing up it was not considered cricket to cry and show your emotions. If you got mad, that was okay. Your old man might let you get away with that, but if you expressed any softer emotions, it wasn't manly.

In recent years it's become okay for men to talk about their feelings, but many men are still reticent about exposing the tender or confusing or unhappy feelings that are normal to both men and women as they go through life.

In fact, some men are so conditioned to the old ideas of manliness that they initially have trouble pinpointing *any* Vital Needs. But those needs are there and can be discovered and acted upon. The Dallas Doctors were somewhat reluctant to talk about their Vital Needs with each other in class, but during the following week each put together a list of five Vital Needs and began the process of more fully incorporating the fulfillment of those needs into daily life.

The Dallas Doctors were pleased with their increased awareness of what is important to them, and they all found that when they made sure to have their Vital Needs met most of the time they were much less likely to be drawn into food binges.

I feel the Vital Needs section of the Dallas Doctors' Diet is very important and urge you to give this element of the diet as much attention as you have the preceding instructions on eating styles.

The Dallas Doctors' Week Four weight losses were:

Dr. Jerry Bane—2 pounds
Dr. Cliff Daniel—3 pounds
Dr. Mike Mendelson—3¼ pounds
Dr. Bill Pirtle—1 pound
Dr. Sandy Reitman—3 pounds
Dr. Jack Wilson—3 pounds

One of the most impressive aspects of this diet is that weekly weight losses are not dangerously high or discouragingly low. The human body is capable of handling a 2- to 4-pound drop in weight each week without difficulty. Endocrine functions won't get out of kilter; electrolyte balances will remain stable; bowel function isn't likely to alter; diet-triggered mood disturbances such as depression, fatigue, and jitteriness aren't likely to occur; skin is not as prone to sagging the way it often does when people lose huge amounts of weight very quickly.

Other diets are more dramatic in their initial weight-loss figures, but most of them are, in my opinion, unhealthy and eventually end up stressing the body twice—once when the weight comes off, and again, when the weight goes back on. It should be comforting to you to know, as you proceed toward your goal weight on the 3D program, that you are achieving healthy, gradual changes that both you and your body can live with.

You have now followed our six Dallas doctors for a month as they dieted in a way that was entirely new to them. As you have seen, they all did well and retained their enthusiasm for the 3D program. The doctors' total weight losses on the One Month Dallas Doctors' Diet program were:

Dr. Jerry Bane—10 pounds
Dr. Cliff Daniel—16 pounds
Dr. Mike Mendelson—17 pounds
Dr. Bill Pirtle—13 pounds
Dr. Sandy Reitman—16 pounds
Dr. Jack Wilson—20 pounds

You will get an up-date on how well Doctors Bane, Daniel, Mendelson, Pirtle, Reitman and Wilson have maintained their weight losses and their present attitudes toward the 3D diet later in this book.

11

EATING OUT: RESTAURANTS, BUFFETS, HOLIDAYS, VACATIONS

MOST DIETERS DREAD eating out. At home you have everything under control. Your refrigerator, stocked with deskinned chicken breasts, celery stalks, diet margarine and low-cal sodas, doesn't lend itself to gluttonous raids. Cupboards are bereft of any inviting packages of crackers, cookies, chips and pretzels. The bread box remains bare.

You are safe. Miserable, but safe.

But the minute that a menu is placed in your hands at any restaurant you know you're in for one of two unhappy experiences—either you pick away forlornly at your steamed fish and salad greens while your dinner companions lap up their crabmeat au gratin and veal parmigiano, or you throw all caution to the winds and

stuff yourself with every fattening food you've longed
for and then you end up hating yourself for having blown
your diet and proved to yourself and the world *again*
that you have no character.

I faced the restaurant dilemma many times during my
years of chronic dieting, which is why I'm so appreciative
of the fact that on my diet you can actually *enjoy* eating
out. You can expect on the 3D diet to be able to go to
any restaurant, choose the items you relish and eat them
without gaining weight.

You will be able to eat in public places just like any
normal-weight person.

IF—

if you eat in the Naturally Slim way that you have been
learning in this book, i.e.,

- eat only when hungry so that Fat-Burn-Out can
take place;
- eat slowly;
- take the five minute breaks;
- avoid Unthinking Food Combinations;
- drink the water;
- eat in order of preference.

I know you have heard Wayne and me give you these
same instructions quite a few times, but my experience
as a teacher has shown me that you cannot remind the
new 3D dieter too often about the basics during the early
weeks on this program.

Dining out can be treacherous in the beginning *only*
if you slip back into your old ways of eating when thrust
into social situations. Unless you stay on guard, you may
start eating at the pace of others at the table. You may

find yourself forgetting to eat in order of preference and eating foods you don't like much just because the old you was used to eating everything the waitress put down in front of you.

Your safeguards against weight gain are these few new eating principles. Follow them and restaurant eating will be the pleasure for you that you deserve.

Buffets also can have their pitfalls. All those tables laden with lavish amounts and varieties of food can escalate you into a temporary state of food mania. There you are, the foodaholic, placed in a room piled high with a dazzling variety of appetizers, main dishes and desserts for you to sample at will. What would the *old* you have done? Gone into sensory overload, grabbed a big plate and piled it high with as many different foods as you could get to stay on the plate.

But the new you, the budding True Thin, knows that there has to be a better way to deal with buffets. You're right. I spent quite a while studying how True Thins eat at such events, and have come up with an eating plan that will enable you to handle buffet eating with ease.

FIRST: Circle the table slowly. Savor the food with your eyes. Notice the colors, textures, shapes, arrangements. Think about how each food would taste if you chose it. Does the shrimp salad have enough shrimp in it to be worthy of your attention? Does the lemon meringue pie look better than the rolls? Is the roast beef rare enough? Do the deviled eggs make your mouth water in anticipation? Are the beans crisp and green? Do you really want that stuffed pepper that on closer observation looks like it's been reheated too many times? Do you hunger for the mound of rice that goes with the chicken à la king? Does the ravioli look marvelous?

SECOND: Circle the table slowly one more time and narrow down your choices. Is the broiled fish a little too overcooked for your taste? The ham steak dried out? The bowl of fresh shrimp on ice enticing?

THIRD: Get a plate and then think, "What is *special?* What will I feel deprived of if I don't have it?" Go right to this food and put it on your plate. If there are one or two items that you feel you must have or you will feel cheated of a full sensory experience, add these foods to your plate.

FOURTH: Take your plate and sit down. Start eating item number one first. When you have finished *all* of it, then move on to the next item and eat as much of it as it takes to feel satisfied, then STOP.

FIFTH: Take a two- to five-minute rest. Talk to someone, or look around at the crowd.

SIXTH: Now think, am I satisfied or do I want to go back for more food? If you are still hungry, it is all right to return to the buffet table, but again, choose only one or two items and take small servings. Eat these selections in the same manner that you did your first helping.

SEVENTH: Think. Do I feel comfortably full? Pleased at what I have eaten? Eaten exactly what I wanted? Good. Then STOP!

EIGHTH: Drink some water, then close your meal with coffee or tea if you so desire.

You have just adapted your old, unselective, fattening

style of eating to a new, quality-eating process. You tailored the buffet to your personal appetite and food tastes and, by giving yourself permission to eat what you want instead of indiscriminately eating everything available to you, you have pampered and rewarded yourself with a memorable food event. That's what TRUE food freedom is all about—the pleasure of eating the best of foods until you're comfortably satiated, in the knowledge that you won't gain weight while doing so.

Holiday eating is a little trickier because you're not dealing with a single food event, but a series of events that are often spread, as in the case of Christmas week, over several days.

Holiday menus tend to be top heavy in the dessert department, and you're constantly being ambushed by boxes of chocolates, plates of fruit cake, platters of homemade cookies, bowls of egg nog and punch, mounds of sugar-coated dried fruits and nuts.

And you're being given FOOD IS LOVE messages: "I made this stollen just for you, because I remember how much you loved it as a child;" "Mama always said, 'No Thanksgiving is complete without Grandma's special candied yams,' so make sure you get a big helping of those yams, now, you hear?" "I stayed up until three in the morning making the mincemeat pies. You're not going to disappoint me and not eat at least one piece, are you?"

Also, many family holiday reunions are emotionally charged, tense affairs, which can trigger emotional eating. Even worse, some holiday gatherings prove to be *boring*, which also can cause you to eat to excess.

All of which doesn't mean that holidays have to be food binge disasters. I have given you the tools to control your eating so that you can achieve maximum pleasure from normal size quantities of food. Use these tools.

During any holiday you can choose to continue to lose weight or maintain that weight. If you decide to maintain, remember that that is not a license to eat as if you are "off your diet," and able to stuff yourself like a Christmas goose!

You are making a responsible decision to expand your eating choices *to some extent,* so that you can enjoy those special foods that are usually available only at holiday time. My HOLIDAY EATING TECHNIQUES should help you avoid overeating.

HOLIDAY EATING TECHNIQUES

1. Holidays and parties are loaded with Unthinking Food Combinations. Ignore them. You are used to thinking that you must eat some of everything presented. Not so! Discover what you want the most and eat that. For example, you know that turkey, gravy, dressing, mashed potatoes, cranberry sauce, peas, creamed onions, hot rolls, fruit salad, sweet potatoes and dessert all come together, but if you want only the dressing, mashed potatoes, gravy, fruit salad and rolls, put the dessert aside for dinner the next day and save the turkey and have it in a sandwich later.

2. Use Save Your Hungers or have a very light snack instead of eating lunch the day of the big dinner, and then you will be at a full HUNGER LEVEL 3 when dinner is served. That way you will be able to eat to fullness and satiety and not pay for it in weight gain.

3. If you should overeat, DON'T PANIC. Just wait until you experience true hunger again before you eat anything else. This will keep you in touch with your true hunger signal and minimize weight gain. For example,

should you overeat Thanksgiving dinner at 2:00 P.M., you may not experience true hunger until 2:00 or 3:00 the next day. Don't let this alarm you. Your body is just taking care of the excess food and that takes time.

4. Don't assume that because it is a holiday you have to talk about food. Eat it and enjoy it, but don't dwell on it.

IF YOU ARE DOING THE COOKING:

1. Quickly select the recipe you are going to use. Don't sidetrack yourself and get your susceptible taste buds aroused by reading other recipes.

2. Go to the grocery store only once . . . at the most, twice.

3. Do not taste while cooking. You can correct the seasonings in the finished product just before serving it (when you are at HUNGER LEVEL 3).

4. Give dishes that cause you temptation or stress to other members of your family to prepare.

5. When each food is prepared, cover it immediately or put it away. "Food sitting out" creates a flirt food situation.

6. If you are taking food to someone else's house, volunteer to bring something that takes little or no time to prepare, such as rolls and butter, wine, plates and napkins, nuts, coffee.

Holidays are meant to be enjoyed on many levels. Work is suspended. You're with people you care about whom you don't get to see much of ordinarily. The religious, traditional or sentimental aspects of the special day should be savored instead of turning the occasion into a food binge. Only perennial dieters approach holidays with the attitude that they must eat everything they see, so they will be stocked up enough to endure the inevitable deprivation diet that is to follow. Now that you are getting into the habit of eating like a True Thin, you should be able to understand and be contented with the fact that this is not the last holiday eating opportunity you will ever have. As a matter of fact, there will be at least *fifty* more holiday/special events like birthdays and anniversaries this year!

Vacation eating should be handled in the same way that you deal with restaurant eating, buffets and holiday spreads. I have one added helpful suggestion to pass on to you that a number of my True Thin friends use to avoid overeating when traveling: instead of trying to eat right then every unique food you want on the theory that you'll never get the opportunity to eat that food again, ship some of those special ethnic and regional delicacies to your home for later enjoyment.

12

HOW TO DEAL WITH THE SABOTEURS

THE BIGGEST HURDLE you will have to overcome on the 3D diet is thinking that if the rest of the family is dining, you have to too or they will be upset. I don't mean to be unkind, but if it bothers family members when you don't eat when they're eating, that's a shame, but it's their problem not yours. Your primary responsibility at the moment is to make yourself comfortable with your new eating "only when hungry" pattern. Your family will weather your not matching them forkful for forkful. You want to lose weight and keep it off forever, right? So you must make it clear to your loved ones that *if they really love you,* they will help you to achieve your goal by removing the pressure to conform to their eating habits instead of your own.

After all, you're not asking them to change any of *their* ways of eating; you only want them not to sabotage *your* efforts to change from an Overeater into a True Thin!

When I first started on my diet, I was afraid that my husband, Justin, would be very upset if I didn't eat dinner when he was ready to eat. I remember the first evening I sat down to dinner when I was at Hunger Level 2. I knew I didn't dare eat yet, so I drank a glass of tea and didn't call attention to the fact that I wasn't eating, and do you know, *no one noticed that I wasn't eating!* You see, because my mouth wasn't full and I wasn't having to chew a lot of food, I was able to fill Justin in on the day's events and talk to the children about their activities.

Then within several weeks, an interesting thing happened. Justin started asking me if I was eating or not eating that night, and it turned out he was more pleased if I *wasn't* eating, because he got more of my attention. It's very important to him that I be at the table, but it's *un*important to him that I always eat when he's eating. What I often do is sip some tea or coffee and enjoy being with him. So my eating only when at Hunger Level 3 has *helped* my marriage rather than hurt it.

I do suggest that when you start my diet you sit your family down and explain to them that you are learning to become a normal-weight person who won't have to diet constantly. Tell them that from now on it will be necessary for you to eat only when you are hungry and you will be eating some foods that they have formerly thought were too fattening for you to eat. Also, explain that since you will be eating very slowly, they don't have to stay at the table with you until you finish your meal if they are through and restless. Also, ask your family not to criticize what you're doing. Your steady weight losses on the 3D program will answer all potential criticism that your family might have.

Keep in mind, too, that trying to synchronize your family's eating schedules with your own will not be a problem forever. As you progress on the 3D diet, you will become adept at using Save Your Hungers to juggle your eating time so that you are at HUNGER LEVEL 3 when the rest of the family is ready to dine.

You are likely to encounter several more saboteurs during the early stages of the 3D diet:

The Nap Trap

You wake up from a lovely nap to find that you're hungry, hungry, hungry. Before, you would have made a beeline for the kitchen and eaten something. Don't be fooled by the Nap Trap. This is *false* hunger. Drink a big, tall glass of water, walk around the house for a few minutes to wake yourself up, and voilà!—you'll find your hunger pangs are gone.

Kind Friends

I don't know why, but the very friends who have urged you to go on a diet are usually the first to sabotage your efforts to *stay* on that diet! They offer you forbidden foods, saying, "Oh, it won't hurt you to eat this just this once." They give you gifts of candy and other sweets because, "I know you like chocolates so much and since I don't eat them I didn't want them to go to waste." Your Kind Friends will also tell you, "Oh, you can always start your diet again tomorrow."

There is no point in trying to educate your Kind Friends or tangling with them. When offered food you don't want, just say, "Thank you. I'm not hungry at the moment, but I would love to take a piece of your beautiful cake (or remaining casserole, or whatever) home with me and eat it later when I'm not too full to enjoy it." Whether you actually do eat it later or not, your Kind Friends will never know, so no feelings will get hurt.

Scary Words

Don't use negative, scary words to describe the positive feeling of being hungry. Such exaggerated descriptions of hunger as, "I'm famished," "I'm ravenous," "I'm starving to death," and "My stomach thinks my throat has been cut," lay the psychological foundation for eating large amounts of food. If you *were* starving to death, then it would make sense to you and everyone else around you for you to really put the food away. But you're *not* starving.

We don't say "I need to go to the bathroom so badly that my bladder will rupture and I'll have to go to the hospital," or, "I'm so tired I'll probably die in my sleep," so don't psych yourself into overeating by using words and phrases like "starving to death." Never use any word but "hungry." It's your best linguistic friend, because it will get and keep you thin.

Food Fascination

Overeaters are susceptible to stimulating themselves into false hunger when they see, hear, smell, taste, talk or read about food. Therefore, until you have reached

your goal weight, I want you to avoid (1) what I call
Food Fascination—reading cookbooks, food ads, recipes,
food magazines—and (2) talking about restaurants and
reminiscing about good and bad meals.

Think about this for a moment. You are still as susceptible to food binging as a newly-on-the-wagon alcoholic
is to alcohol. An alcoholic would be putting himself in
a dangerous position if he or she talked about drinks and
drinking right then. It wouldn't make any sense for an
alcoholic to gaze at books showing drinks and the recipes
for making them or to bring liquor to a party or to volunteer to be the bartender at a party. Like the newly recov-
ered alcoholic, you want to avoid tempting yourself unduly until your body has had a chance to reestablish
healthy eating patterns and you have become accustomed
to these new patterns. Once you've reached the weight
you wish to stay at, then you can play with Food Fascination again, for you will be strong enough to handle it.

Loose Clothes

Loose clothes encourage you to eat past fullness, so
throw your "fat" clothes away or have them altered immediately once you begin to lose weight on the 3D diet.
Since you are becoming a True Thin, you can now take
advantage of one of their techniques to help them maintain their weight. True Thins wear snug clothes and if
those clothes become unpleasantly tight, they cut back
on their food intake for a few days until their wardrobe
is once more comfortable to wear. Believe me, it is very
hard to overeat when you are wearing a pair of blue
jeans that fit you like the paper on the wall! So get out
of those baggy "comfits" that were part of your fat past

and tuck yourself into trim, tight clothes that will be more helpful in getting you to your True Thin future.

Scales

Many Overeaters weigh themselves all the time. Most True Thins don't even have scales in their homes, or if they do, they are probably stored in the garage because they weigh inaccurately! True Thins don't need scales because they don't fluctuate much in weight. Overeaters have *many* ups and downs, as you are all too well aware, and they react badly to those ups. Normal-weight people just cut back on their food for a short time when they see that they have put on a few pounds; overweight people get so depressed that they eat even more than usual, send their weight soaring, confirm the latest eating disaster on the scales and then, that's right . . . they eat some more.

Since you are a card-carrying Overeater you are prone to overreacting to weigh-ins, so I want you to stay off the scales during the first month of the Dallas Doctors' Diet program. Obviously, you will be intensely curious about just how much weight you are losing, so it will be all right if you weigh yourself ONCE EVERY EIGHT DAYS . . . but no more. Why not every seven days? Because on the 3D diet, for reasons I don't fully understand, your true weight losses will show up on the scale in eight-day increments. I also recommend that you do your weighing-in immediately after awakening.

You will probably want to keep a running record of your weight losses. I suggest that you write your current weight on your weekly Food Sheets, at the top of the first day's sheet.

Also, weigh in on the same scale each time, and use accurate scales. If you don't own a good one and don't want to invest in a new one, your doctor might let you weigh in on one of the several he keeps correctly calibrated in his examining rooms; or you might check out the accuracy of the large scale that many supermarkets keep in the entrances of the stores for the convenience of shoppers. Most of the supermarket scales I have tested have been surprisingly accurate and have the added advantage, for those of you who are severely obese, of being able to register higher poundage than most home scales.

13

IF THE DIET DOESN'T SEEM TO BE WORKING FOR YOU

THE SEVERAL THOUSAND people who have gone through Sandra Breithaupt's Naturally Slim program have had one advantage over you, the reader. Whenever they found the instructions confusing, or if those instructions didn't seem to work for them, they were able to consult with the course instructor and get their individual problem solved.

I cannot give you the highly personalized answers that a course instructor would give; however, I believe that I can offer solutions to several difficulties that have been encountered in this diet by class members. There are two sets of problems—"I'm not losing any weight," and, "I'm not losing as much weight as I would like to."

Let's look at the first complaint—"I'm not losing any weight." There have been a few, very few, people who have failed to take off any weight, despite the fact that they have followed the principles of this diet to the letter; they have eaten only when at HUNGER LEVEL 3, drunk their 60 ounces of water a day, eaten slowly, etc. We have been able to trace these people's problem to the fact that they were taking medications that interfered with their body's ability to achieve daily Fat-Burn-Out. Any of the following families of medications can partially block your ability to lose weight:

- birth-control pills
- steroids
- anti-depressant drugs
- anti-inflammatory drugs
- hormones used to treat certain gynecologic disorders

Weight gain is only a *potential* side effect of various prescription drugs. Please be clear that I am NOT saying that all people who take such medications will be unable to lose weight on diets. I am only pointing out that if you have not lost weight on the 3D diet, there is a possibility that medications being taken by you could be blocking your body's ability to shed fat. DON'T STOP TAKING ANY DRUG THAT YOUR PHYSICIAN HAS PRESCRIBED FOR YOU! Instead, consult with him about the possibility of changing to another medication within the same family of drugs that does not have weight gain as a side effect.

For those of you saying, "I'm not losing as much weight as I would like to," I have several clues to why this could be so:

1. You may be drinking alcoholic beverages at HUN-GER LEVEL 2 instead of waiting until you have reached HUNGER LEVEL 3.

2. Your diet may be top heavy in cheese. A small percentage of people who consume large amounts of cheese and other dairy foods will slow down or stop their Fat-Burn-Out. So while you're dieting, I recommend that you avoid eating cheese dishes more than once a week. When you reach your goal weight, you may add more cheese to your menus if you wish to.

3. Cereal can also slow down your Fat-Burn-Out mechanism, so I suggest that you curtail your intake of commercial, packaged dry cereals. You may, however, continue to add bran to foods if you usually do so, to increase the amount of fiber in your diet.

4. You may still be eating *past* fullness. If you have been used to eating big portions in the past, your eye could be deceiving your stomach. I suggest that this week you stop eating before you think you are quite full and see if this doesn't tip the scales in your favor. There are several ways to make stopping eating early easier for you:

    a. chew a piece of gum . . .

    b. sip a beverage . . .

    c. have a small piece of fruit . . .

    d. eat six peanuts . . .

    e. eat one teaspoon of peanut butter . . .

    f. move your plate to a different place on the table . . .

    g. cover your plate with your napkin . . .

    h. eat one or two mints . . .

    i. put your plate in the dishwasher . . .

    j. put on lipstick . . .

    k. brush your teeth.

5. You may be so schooled to not overeat that you are failing to eat *enough* food at each meal! If you don't eat to fullness, you will find yourself eating, for example, three meals a day when you actually have two-time-a-day hunger and should be eating twice a day; or you could be eating twice a day when you are a one-time-a-day hunger person. Always eat enough food to feel really satiated.

6. Most overweight people are so unfamiliar with the feeling of hunger that they mistake appetite for hunger. If you are not attaining a satisfactory weight loss, you may be eating at HUNGER LEVEL 2 or HUNGER LEVEL 2½ instead of waiting until you have reached HUNGER LEVEL 3.

7. You may not be drinking all the water advised. Some people use gimmicks to make sure they take in 60 ounces a day, such as placing six glasses in the refrigerator each morning so that they can tell without thinking how many they have drunk by the number of glasses left on the shelf.

You might paint a stripe around a plastic jug or other container at the 60-ounce level. When I first began the 3D diet I decided to drink the six glasses of water at approximately the same times each day so that I wouldn't have to remember whether I had drunk one or two glasses so far that morning. I still pretty much follow my original plan, which was to drink one glass of water upon awakening, another after morning surgery, a third before lunch, the fourth at 4:00 P.M., the fifth just before dinner, and the last one before retiring for the night. In actuality, water drinking has become such a habit with me now that I drink more than the required 60 ounces a day because I've learned to like the taste of water.

There is no question that the water is an important factor in achieving high weight losses on this diet. I did a little two-week controlled experiment to satisfy my own curiosity on this matter. I ate exactly the same foods each day in the same quantity each of those weeks. The only variable was that one week I drank 60 ounces of water per day, the other I didn't. The week without the water, I lost half a pound. The week I drank all the water, I lost a little under *four pounds*. I am convinced that your success will be much greater when you drink all the water.

8. Another habit that can slow down your weight loss is eating too many diet foods. Perennial dieters have developed a self-punishing mentality about weight-loss programs. They associate all diets with suffering and expect to have to eat only foods they don't like while they are in their self-imposed diet prison. Such people divide all foods into Should and Shouldn't categories, Should foods being low-calorie, dull foods, Shouldn't foods being the wonderful ones they eat only when they are being "bad."

If you have been separating food into Should/Shouldn't categories, I want you to stop. One of the tenets of this diet is that you must eat only foods that are pleasurable to you. If you happen to feel you'd be willing to fight for water-packed tuna, dressingless salads, dry-boiled fish, and cottage cheese and the like, fine. But I seriously doubt that diet foods are your favorite ones, or you wouldn't be overweight. When you start eating those Shouldn't foods you love, your weight losses will be higher, because you will be satisfied with smaller quantities of food and you won't be fighting feelings of wanting to flee being in a diet prison. Such feelings can push you into eating before you reach HUNGER LEVEL 3 and cause you to be easily ensnared by flirt food situations.

The Dallas Doctors' Diet is not a temporary, punishing diet. It is a rewarding new way of eating that I hope you will stay with for the rest of your life. If you choose pleasurable foods as your daily staples, you will soon shed your diet prison mentality and with it unsatisfactory weight losses.

9. Attitude is another factor in how quickly you will lose weight. Are you the kind of person who sees only ways you *can't* do things? If so, you will have a difficult time on this diet. Do you tell yourself, "I *can't* drink all that water," "I *can't* cook without tasting," "I *can't* refuse food when it's offered to me because I'll hurt people's feelings," "I *can't* sit at the same table with others who are eating and not eat with them," "I *can't* eat only at HUNGER LEVEL 3 because family, friends and business associates expect me to adjust to their schedules"? Unless you can acknowledge that your "I can'ts" are mental blocks that *you* have set up so that you can stay in your familiar fat world, you won't be able to achieve satisfactory weight losses on this program.

Any of the nine explanations in this chapter could be the missing key to your taking off your excess weight and keeping that weight off. It has been my observation, however, that the main reason 20% of the people who go on the 3D (or any other diet) program fail, is that they are not motivated to lose weight.

You could be liking the idea of being thin, and feeling guilty about being overweight, or worried about the health risks endemic to obesity, but still not be *ready* to make the major adjustments in your eating habits that will be necessary to change from being an Overeater to a True Thin.

You should also consider the possibility, if the 3D diet isn't working for you, that you don't want to be thin. If so, no diet is going to be successful. Many people who really don't want to be well suffer from illnesses of all kinds. This is a subconscious phenomenon, one they are usually unaware of. We have several sayings in the "doctor trade" that describe this. One is "Hardly a day goes by that we don't have someone come in the office looking for a disease." Another is, "He (or she) has been enjoying his poor health for so long that he is not about to let us get him well." These are generally people whose lives are so empty that having some sort of malady is mandatory for survival.

Let me give you a recent example. A year ago one of my patients came in for her annual exam, and during the visit we discussed her overweight problem, which was a significant one. I explained the Naturally Slim program with all of its virtues and encouraged her to call Ruth Thomas, the program's instructor, for further details. A year went by and she returned for her physical checkup having gained a few more pounds. I inquired if she had looked into taking the course and she said she had. But then she stated that she had discovered from talking to many people that the system really worked and that they *had* lost weight and were not having trouble maintaining their weight loss!

"Well," I asked, "What's the problem?" After a few seconds of serious thought, she said, "If I had taken the course and was successful and lost to a normal weight, then what would I do?" In other words, she had enough insight into herself to know that her obesity was serving some purpose. With success, be it financial or in some other area of our lives, comes responsibility. Unfortunately, some people choose, knowingly or unknowingly, to be unsuccessful. It's important for your own peace of mind to know if you are psychologically able to diet at this moment so that you can accept or discard lack of motivation as a reason for the 3D diet's not meeting your expectations.

There's no such thing as being a little bit pregnant, or a little bit on the 3D program. Either your desire to be thin is strong enough to commit you to a course of action or it isn't. If not, don't try this diet, because you will fail in it, as you have in all the other diets you have hazarded when you weren't ready emotionally to give up your old ways of eating.

Just because you're not motivated to become a True Thin now, doesn't mean that you will have to spend the rest of your life fat. The very fact that you have read this far into the book means that you are already committed enough to the prospect of dieting to *consider* ways of losing weight. This is a hopeful beginning.

Perhaps in the not too distant future you will resolve the personal problems in your life that are blocking your ability to be a normal-weight person. If this does happen, I would recommend that you give the 3D diet a chance, as this program is the only one available, to my knowledge, that will allow you a high degree of emotional satiety through food.

For those of you who *are* motivated at this moment to lose your excess weight once and for all, I have a suggestion that should help you keep your resolve and success rate high: organize a support group of equally overweight friends and neighbors, and all of you go on the Dallas

Doctors' Diet program together. The initial confusions and adjustments in eating habits will be easier to handle if you share your experiences with a support group. The six Dallas Doctors in this book were unanimous in their opinion that being able to meet with each other once a week helped keep them motivated to stick to the diet and made dieting more fun.

14

THE MOST FREQUENTLY ASKED QUESTIONS

Q. There is no mention of exercise in this book. Isn't exercise important?

DR. AGNEW. *Exercise is very definitely important to long-term health, and I strongly recommend a regular, sensible exercise program. The reason we haven't stressed this is that whether or not you exercise won't affect your ability to change from an Overeater to a True Thin. Also, there are already a number of very fine exercise books in print that cover the subject thoroughly. If you wish to start an exercise program while you are on the 3D diet, I recommend your investigating Dr. Kenneth Cooper's various books on aerobics, Bonnie Pruden's* How to Keep Slender And Fit After Thirty *and* Fit or Fat, *by Covert Bailey.*

Q. How long do I have to keep filling in the daily Food Sheets?

SANDRA BREITHAUPT. *For six weeks. After that you can make up your own mind about whether you feel the information that can be gleaned from your Food Sheets is still helpful. I find that Food Sheets can be very useful barometers of whether you are continuing to eat enough exciting foods, if you are drinking the water recommended, taking the five-minute breaks, eating enough nutritious foods, and controlling your intake of sweets.*

Some people like to do a week of Food Sheets every few months just to reinforce the basic principles of the 3D diet. Others go back to Food Sheets only during a week when they are taking off fluff pounds.

Q. What are fluff pounds?

S.B. *Fluff pounds are those two or three pounds you put on because of special occasion eating that gets out of hand. I call them fluff pounds because it describes them so perfectly. They come off easily—generally with two days of applying every principle of the program again. Fluff pounds will disappear immediately if you tackle them within seventy-two hours of their showing up on the scales.*

Q. Can I go on the 3D diet while I am pregnant?

DR. A. *I wouldn't recommend that you do so, for you should be gaining weight, not losing it during your months of pregnancy. A healthy increase would be approximately one-half pound per week during the first half of your pregnancy, and one pound during the second half. You should also be particularly careful to eat balanced, nutritious meals during this special time. I suppose that someone who has already*

*been through the Naturally Slim program could tai-
lor its principles to her pregnancy, but otherwise
the mother-to-be might be better served by waiting
until she is post partum to start this or any diet.*

Q. When will the plateaus hit?

S.B. *They won't hit. There are no "dry spells" when
you can't get the scales to budge on the 3D program.
The degree to which you are overweight, however,
will affect the rapidity of your weight loss. People
who are only moderately overweight lose weight
much more quickly than those who are obese.*

Q. Won't drinking all that water and not eating three
meals a day produce vitamin and mineral deficien-
cies?

DR. A. *We have not seen any cases of a large water
intake "washing" vitamins and minerals out of the
system; nor will failing to eat three meals a day cause
malnutrition. But if you are accustomed to taking
a vitamin supplement or feel you need it, by all
means go ahead and take a daily all-purpose vita-
min/mineral supplement.*

Q. My stomach "growls" if I don't eat breakfast. Doesn't
that mean I'm hungry and should eat?

DR. A. *No. A "growling" or "rumbling" sound is not
a sign of hunger and, in actuality, the sound you
describe is not coming from the stomach, which sits
predominantly behind the lower ribs, but from the
intestines in your abdominal cavity. Food moves
through your intestines by means of bursts of peri-
staltic waves and rhythmic contractions of segments
of the intestine, and it's that movement of food
through the intestines that causes the growling/rum-
bling sounds (called borborygmi) that many people*

assume are hunger pangs. Ignore them. They aren't signs that it's time to eat.

Q. How many weeks can I stay on this diet?

S.B. *As many weeks as it takes to reach your goal weight.*

Q. What should I do when I reach goal weight? Is there a maintenance program?

S.B. *Yes, and it's a very simple one. Just continue with your new Naturally Slim eating habits, but give yourself a bit more leeway. You can eat at hunger Level 2 from time to time. At this point you will be able to "cheat" a little without penalty. Your guides to how well you are doing will be (1) that your clothes don't start feeling tight and (2) you don't show any rise in weight when you get on the scales.*

Earlier in the program I asked you to weigh yourself only every eight days. When you reach maintenance, I want you to weigh much more often so that you can keep a close eye on any fluff pounds and get rid of them before they turn into hard fat.

Q. Will I ever be able to eat cereal again?

S.B. *Yes. After the first month, there are no forbidden foods or beverages.*

Q. If I develop a problem on this diet that I can't find the answer for in this book, will you advise me personally?

DR. A. and S.B. *It would be our pleasure to answer any reader inquiry on how to make the 3D diet work at peak efficiency. Just send your question to us, c/o McGraw-Hill Book Company, 1221 Avenue of the Americas, New York, New York 10020. Enclose a self-addressed, stamped envelope, and you will receive a speedy answer from us.*

15

THE DALLAS DOCTORS ONE YEAR LATER

DR. JERRY BANE

DR. BANE REACHED his weight-loss goal of 21 pounds, and has continued to maintain that weight during this succeeding year. His opinion of the 3D program?

"I never had lasting success with a diet program until I started on the 3D diet. And I'll be honest, I found it strange at first. Very different. This is because I grew up in a family that had three big meals every day. I had never heard anybody say, 'Hey, you don't have to eat just because it's *noon!*' I was kind of intrigued by that. Actually, I still pretty much eat three meals a day because that turned out to be my normal pattern; but I eat differently now in that I don't eat as much, and there are times now when I'm not hungry and I just don't eat.

"Now like all people I kind of slide a little bit, and sometimes I follow the program better than others, but you get it ingrained into you because it's so easy and natural to do. Patients come in and ask me about this diet and that diet, screwy things they've read about someplace, and I recommend the 3D Naturally Slim to them. If for some reason they aren't interested in it, I'll mention Weight Watchers, because I have seen that diet work well on a temporary basis, but I think the 3D diet beats that all to pieces. This is something you can get comfortable with and stay with. One of our biggest problems today is obesity, and anything that controls this in a sane, sensible manner is fantastic, so I'm very enthusiastic about the results that are possible on this diet. My whole family now follows its principles."

DR. CLIFF DANIEL

Dr. Daniel lost 16 pounds and has not regained any of that weight. He continues to eat the 3D way. His overview now, one year later, is:

"The 3D diet was quite a change for me. I was surprised at how very little food it takes to get full on if you eat slower and savor each bite. The most remarkable aspect of the diet to me was that I lost weight while eating a great *variety* of foods. Before, I had always been tied to low-calorie foods, consciously or unconsciously. I'd choose low-calorie foods almost every time. But I don't think I ate *anything* with few calories in it the whole time I was on the 3D. Just smaller quantities. I thought it was a terrific liberation when I sat down and ate a bunch of bread. I'd never been permitted to do that on other diets.

"One of the great things about the 3D is that it helps you break the pattern of 'rewarding yourself' with good things to eat, and feeling guilty afterwards. I think that's kind of left over from our old ideas about dieting (If I'm good, I get to have this baked Alaska). What we have to do, if we are to defeat obesity, is get a sense of satisfying ourselves and making the sensation of hunger go away. In a culture as affluent as ours, you should certainly enjoy food, but it should not be a primary reward mechanism. I think that's really a central point of this program—that food is for sustenance. Only rarely should we use it for entertainment.

"I don't question the diet medically. It makes a lot of sense to wait until you're hungry to eat. That's a lot better than eating on somebody else's schedule. And the 3D works a lot better than fasting if your goal is simply to lose weight quickly. I've fasted before. I've eaten nothing but lettuce before. I've done all these things, but I've *never* lost weight at the rate I lost on this diet.

"One other facet of the program that impressed me is that the diet tends to take away the anxiety associated with losing weight. You don't feel much tension because you know, when you get ready to eat, you're going to eat whatever pleases you.

"Even if you fall off, it's a pattern that's really welcome to get back to. I think the 3D diet is an excellent program."

DR. MIKE MENDELSON

Dr. Mendelson lost a total of 22 pounds on the 3D program, but he gained half of it back during the year, because he slipped back into his old habit of eating too fast. He points out though, that "I'm not eating the quantity I was before, and the diet has helped me arrest my pattern of yearly weight *gain.* I only wish that my group had gone on, for the esprit de corps was nice. Also, as long as I was attending the sessions, I would have been ashamed to go back to my old ways.

"My wife says that I don't really want to lose weight, that I'm happy being 'my chubby self,' and she may be right. However, I am *very,* I mean *very,* resistant to getting any heavier. In fact, I'm pretty much back on the 3D diet at the moment—drinking the water, eating slowly, watching not to eat for emotional reasons.

"The most important aspect of the 3D for me is the idea of eating all kinds of foods, the foods you want, having a large variety without stuffing yourself. It shows that by *intellectually* looking at what you're doing with food, you can really eat anything you want if you do this in a sensible way. I *like* this diet."

DR. BILL PIRTLE

Dr. Pirtle has had no trouble maintaining his weight loss since finishing the 3D course, and continues to be an advocate of the program:

"I was impressed with the program from the very beginning. The slow eating, knowing the difference between appetite and hunger, the chewing your food, the satiety center in the hypothalamus—the whole ball of wax. It was all very significant, and it all fit into place. I feel that understanding about your Vital Needs is what sustains you once you've reached your goal, but I wouldn't really want to single out any one thing. The whole program sustains you, thanks to the habits you develop.

"Most of the overweight people I see in my practice have some type of emotional problem. There's a divorce. They're depressed. The kids are driving them crazy. Their husbands are running around on them or the husband never touches 'em when he comes home. Something is going on in their lives. It's very difficult for them to lose weight, because eating is practically the only enjoyment they get out of life. The sexual relationship may be zero, they're bored with their work, they wish the kids were somewhere else, but eating is still enjoyable. You take that away from them, you put them on one of those real strict diets, those boring diets—man, you'll destroy that individual.

"The 3D program is one that these people can actually live with. You're not going to solve their marital problems. With this program, people can still enjoy the foods they like and need emotionally and, if they follow the rules and give it a little time, they'll lose weight. That's why this diet has a high success rate. I now refer people to the 3D diet. For myself, I am very pleased with the results I have achieved and intend to continue the program."

DR. SANDY REITMAN

Dr. Reitman reports that "my previous exuberance for the program persists, and my weight has remained comfortably stable. The concept of the program is brilliant in its simplicity, and so physiologically sound, in my opinion, that it represents a truly safe approach to weight reduction.

"Before, I always relegated my dieting to times when I wasn't under stress, or when everything was going okay, my practice was great, whatever. And you know, there are hardly ever times like that. Very rarely do grown-up people have wonderful times when they can go on a diet without stress or distraction. The 3D afforded me the opportunity to do it during the regular times, with the parties, the stresses. That is really the only practical way to do it. There is no 'perfect time' to stop smoking, no 'perfect time' to stop eating. It doesn't exist. You have to incorporate weight loss into everyday life. Today, when I'm under stress, I still eat, I don't miss my meals, but I don't eat tremendous quantities like I used to. I can face anything except the most dire circumstances and I still eat in my new pattern.

"My wife, Margaret, thinks the 3D diet is wonderful because I don't complain and suffer anymore, and because it broke me of the habit of turning into a bear at a minute after six if the table wasn't set. She enjoys the devil out of that. Margaret has always eaten 'naturally slim,' but for twenty years I was adamant about dinner time at six o'clock. It was a religious thing with me. But now we're eating the way Margaret has always wanted to eat, and the way I *should* be eating according to the program: when we're hungry. Sometimes we eat at bizarre times, but that's terrific, for having learned to read my hunger signals correctly means that I now have the basis for eating the foods I want and remaining slim for the rest of my life."

DR. JACK WILSON

Dr. Wilson weighs less today than he did when he was in high school. "I can't remember ever being under two hundred pounds and I'm very excited about it. I'm still losing a pound and a half to two pounds a week and I can drink margaritas on the weekend and go eat nachos.

"I don't think I'll ever change my habits back again to what they were. My birthday was Monday, so I had to go to my mother's Sunday and have the big dinner; but I stopped after one helping of all the stuff I used to eat three platefuls of. Monday was my actual birthday, so everybody brought their favorite dishes to the office party, and I tried every one; and then that night my wife made my favorite dish and we had chocolate cake and I said, 'Look, this is my birthday and I'm going to eat it and forget it,' and Tuesday morning I was right back on the diet. I'd gained about a pound and I've lost that since then.

"Being in control is the whole key to the program for me. I can't have somebody say, 'You can't, you can't, you can't.' It doesn't work for me. It's better to say, 'Here are the guidelines, now you choose what you think you want to take responsibility for.' The program is a thinking man or woman's program, and because of that I've found the 3D diet is the easiest and the most natural way to lose weight that I could ever hope to discover.

"I'm sold."

AFTERWORD

WHAT HAS BEEN presented in this book is a system, program, a philosophy, call it what you will, that will allow you to lose weight and keep it off without suffering the stress and tears that you've learned to accept as normal on other diet programs.

We know that the 3D diet works for the vast majority of people who make an honest effort to change to this new style of handling food intake. We may not be able to explain all the reasons why the 3D program works from a purely scientific point of view, for we still know relatively little about the physiological causes of all obesity problems; but it is clear from the sheer numbers of people who have been through the Naturally Slim program, that tuning into, and acting upon, your natural hunger patterns will enable most Overeaters to become True Thins.

We hope you will choose to experience the pleasures and adventures and the rewards that are an integral part of this revolutionary new diet. Weight doesn't have to be an aggravation or humiliation in your life. You can now solve your obesity problem and get on with living.

The world is a wonderful, exciting place to be in, fat or thin, but we believe that, given the choice, you would prefer to be a True Thin. If so, The Dallas Doctors' Diet is the book and the program that can transform your dream of being a thin person into life-long reality. Good luck!

Sandra Breithaupt
Dr. Wayne Agnew

NATURALLY SLIM GLOSSARY

APPETITE. Mental desire for certain foods or foods cooked a specific way. Operates twenty-four hours a day. What you love to eat.

CLOCK-DICTATED EATING. Eating because the clock . . . not your body . . . tells you to eat.

COMFORT LEVEL. Exact moment your stomach has enough food and does not need more.

DEPRIVATION PERSONALITY. Hostile, irritable disposition expressed when favorite foods are prohibited. Also accompanied by a pinched look in the face.

DIETER. An Overeater who changes from high-calorie foods to low-calorie foods. Usually exhibits a "deprivation personality."

209

DIET HABIT.   Going on a diet . . . losing weight . . . then regaining the weight . . . then dieting again. Constant internal hassle about what will be eaten.

FALSE HUNGER.   The feeling of wanting food when the body has no need of nourishment. Can be the result of (1) not drinking water, (2) the natural hunger cycle being disturbed because of eating when not hungry, (3) needing to get Vital Needs met.

FAT-BURN-OUT.   The natural ability of the body to eliminate excess fat. Only functions at peak efficiency when food is eaten during true hunger . . . or LEVEL 3.

FLIRT FOODS.   Those foods that appeal to you when you *see* them . . . but you do not even think of them before you see them. They leave your mind as soon as you get away from them. Examples: Doughnuts with the coffee, and candy at a check-out stand.

FOOD FASCINATION.   Overemphasis on food. Using food as the topic of reading material. Using food as the topic of conversations. Using food to structure time. Examples: reading cookbooks like novels; talking about recipes; talking about what you are going to eat . . . what you ate . . . and where are the best places to eat.

GOBBLER.   A person who chews food superfast . . . and reaches for the next bite before even swallowing the first bite. A person who treats eating as an activity to be done with speed.

HUNGER.   Need of the body for nourishment.

HUNGER LEVEL 1.   No hunger.

HUNGER LEVEL 2.   Some hunger. The time to plan the food you will want to eat when you experience full hunger . . . LEVEL 3. YOUR BODY BURNS THE MOST FAT BETWEEN LEVEL 2 AND LEVEL 3.

HUNGER LEVEL 3. True hunger time when the body will burn off fat; and the time when you can eat what you please and not gain weight.

HUNGER LEVEL 4. Ravenous hunger. You are so hungry you will eat past the point of satiety.

HYPOTHALAMUS. A part of the brain which contains the appetite and fullness response centers. From the time you begin to eat it takes twenty minutes or longer for the appetite and fullness centers to register. Both centers should register for you to be able to stop eating and feel satisfied but not stuffed.

MORNING HUNGER PERSON. A person who *daily* has *full* hunger upon awakening (LEVEL 3).

NATURALLY SLIM. A person who has achieved normal weight using methods natural to the body. Goal weight can be maintained with ease.

NATURALLY SLIM INC. The six-week course whose basic tenets were incorporated into this book.

OVEREATER. A person who *daily* eats "when not hungry." The food eaten when not hungry may be a small amount or a large amount.

SATIETY CENTER. Center in your hypothalamus that registers when you satisfy your appetite. Does not register complete satisfaction unless you eat what you want . . . thus making you want more food even though you are full.

SHOULD AND SHOULDN'T FOODS. The foods you have been told you should or shouldn't eat as long as you have a weight problem. Only dieters have these categories in their head.

SAVE YOUR HUNGER. A tiny quantity of food used when experiencing full hunger (LEVEL 3) to "tide you over" and keep you comfortable when you want to wait until a while later to eat. NOT snacking!

Recommended Quantities

6 peanuts........12 halves

or

½ ounce of cheese......cut in small pieces (suck it)

or

1 teaspoon of creamy peanut butter....slowly licked

SWEET CLOSURE. 50 calories of a sweet eaten at the conclusion of a meal to "finish up."

SWEET EXPERIENCE. Sweet that can be eaten once a week in the place of a meal. Never to exceed 500 calories.

THINKING FOOD COMBINATION. Two or more foods eaten together because you purposefully choose to combine them. EACH FOOD IS EXACTLY WHAT YOU REALLY WANT.

THINKING FOOD. A food that is especially appealing to you at a *certain* time. The same food may not be as appealing at another time.

TRUE THIN. A person who has never had a weight problem. Such people cannot understand why you have a problem weighing what you want to weigh. Since you eat so often . . . they assume you have a *lot* of *hunger*. True Thins usually eat only when they are at HUNGER LEVEL 3, but occasionally, when an especially appealing food . . . something they really want to eat . . . is offered to them they may eat it even if they aren't hungry. But they will then return to their hunger cues. They do not do this on a regular basis. True Thins differ from Overeaters in that they think eating only when hungry is normal.

UNTHINKING FOOD COMBINATION. Two or more foods eaten together . . . without thinking if *each* food is *really* what you want at that time. You may *like* each food in the combination, but you do not *intensely* want each food in the combination. Unthinking food combinations cause overeating . . . weight gain . . . dissatisfaction from meals. Examples: cultural combinations: salad, baked potato, steak, roll, crackers.

VITAL NEEDS. Your own individual needs from society and from your personal environment. These needs must be met to have a sense of well-being. When needs are not met . . . overeating can result.

WATER. The single substance of greatest nutritional value to man. The body must have intracellular water to enable it to burn fat efficiently and rapidly. We constantly lose water through (1) respiration (2) perspiration (3) evaporation (4) urination. This water must be consistently replaced for us to stay properly hydrated.

TEA acts as a diuretic and cannot be substituted for your water on this program.

COFFEE acts as a diuretic and cannot be substituted for your water on this program.

LACK OF SUFFICIENT WATER (WE FIND) CAUSES OVEREATERS TO EXPERIENCE "FALSE HUNGER" . . . TO *THINK* THEY WANT FOOD.

INDEX